Recent Scientific and Therapeutic Advances in Allograft

Edited by Norihide Fukushima

Published in London, United Kingdom

Recent Scientific and Therapeutic Advances in Allograft
http://dx.doi.org/10.5772/intechopen.107729
Edited by Norihide Fukushima

Contributors
Adnane Wardani, Alisher Ismailbaev, Anneke Farías-Yapur, Asad Ullah, Estela Azeka, Khalid AlMeshari, Laurence Evrard, Madonna Lee, Mikhail D. Nuzhdin, Nikita Bashmakov, Roman N. Komarov, Sadaki Asari, Shinichi Matsumoto, Takumi Fukumoto, Vladimir A. Bolsunovsky, Yoshihide Nanno

First published in London, United Kingdom, 2024 by IntechOpen
IntechOpen is the global imprint of INTECHOPEN LIMITED, registered in England and Wales, registration number: 11086078, 5 Princes Gate Court, London, SW7 2QJ, United Kingdom
Printed in Croatia

British Library Cataloguing-in-Publication Data
A catalogue record for this book is available from the British Library

Additional hard and PDF copies can be obtained from orders@intechopen.com

Recent Scientific and Therapeutic Advances in Allograft
Edited by Norihide Fukushima
p. cm.

This title is part of the Biomedical Engineering Book Series, Volume 22
Topic: Biotechnology - Biosensors, Biomaterials and Tissue Engineering
Series Editor: Robert Koprowski
Topic Editor: Luis Jesús Villarreal-Gómez

Print ISBN 978-1-83769-129-6
Online ISBN 978-1-83769-130-2
eBook (PDF) ISBN 978-1-83769-131-9
ISSN 2631-5343

IntechOpen Book Series
Biomedical Engineering
Volume 22

Aims and Scope of the Series

Biomedical Engineering is one of the fastest-growing interdisciplinary branches of science and industry. The combination of electronics and computer science with biology and medicine has improved patient diagnosis, reduced rehabilitation time, and helped to facilitate a better quality of life. Nowadays, all medical imaging devices, medical instruments, or new laboratory techniques result from the cooperation of specialists in various fields. The series of Biomedical Engineering books covers such areas of knowledge as chemistry, physics, electronics, medicine, and biology. This series is intended for doctors, engineers, and scientists involved in biomedical engineering or those wanting to start working in this field.

Meet the Series Editor

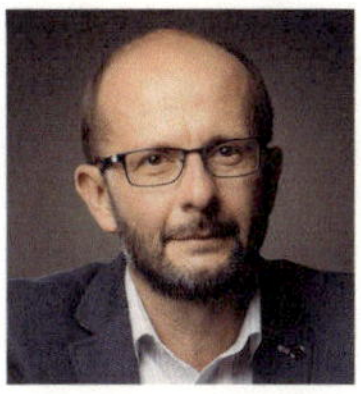

Robert Koprowski, MD (1997), Ph.D. (2003), Habilitation (2015), is an employee of the University of Silesia, Poland, Institute of Computer Science, Department of Biomedical Computer Systems. For 20 years, he has studied the analysis and processing of biomedical images, emphasizing the full automation of measurement for a large inter-individual variability of patients. Dr. Koprowski has authored more than a hundred research papers with dozens in impact factor (IF) journals and has authored or co-authored six books. Additionally, he is the author of several national and international patents in the field of biomedical devices and imaging. Since 2011, he has been a reviewer of grants and projects (including EU projects) in biomedical engineering.

Meet the Volume Editor

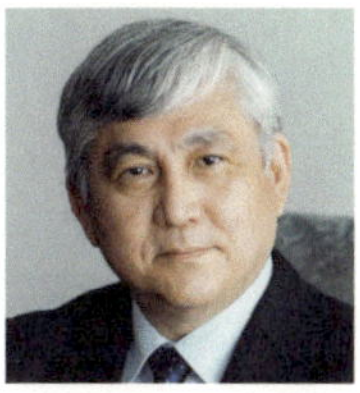

Dr. Norihide Fukushima is a professor at and the president of the Graduate School of Nursing, Senri Kinran University, Japan. He is also a visiting director at the National Cerebral and Cardiovascular Center and a recruit professor in the Department of Surgery, Osaka University Graduate School of Medicine, Japan. After graduating from Osaka University Medical School, Dr. Fukushima completed clinical training in the 1st Department of Surgery, Osaka University Hospital and obtained his Ph.D. in prolonged cardiac immerse storage in 1992. He worked at Loma Linda University, California, USA as a research and clinical fellow from 1991 to 1994. He studied the long-term survival of allogeneic heart transplant goats after a 24-hour immersed preservation technique and concordant (Rhesus monkey to baboon) and discordant (pig to baboon) cardiac xenotransplantation. His team performed the first heart transplantation in Japan in 1999. He and his colleagues revised the Transplant Act in 2010 to increase deceased organ donation and heart transplantation in Japan. He has been working to develop therapeutic strategies for advanced heart failure, such as mechanical circulatory support and medical care.

Contents

Preface

Allograft is a medical procedure in which there is a transfer of cells, tissues, or organs between genetically nonidentical members of the same species. Allografts are commonly used in the transplants of skin, corneas, hearts, lungs, liver, pancreas, kidneys, and bone and bone marrow, although transplants of the latter often come from relatives.

Allograft transplants have been done for more than 150 years, and during this time the processes for ensuring safety have developed. Allograft transplants are becoming increasingly common, with around 2 or 3 million done every year worldwide.

Transplant material is obtained from a donor who is a living person, a deceased person's body receiving mechanical support or ventilation, or a deceased person's body whose heart has stopped beating. Screening for pathology and risk factors for communicable diseases such as HIV and hepatitis B and C is then conducted.

The use of allogeneic (nonself) cells, tissue, and organs carries a high risk of immune rejection and therefore requires tissue matching between donor and recipient. It also involves the administration of immunosuppressive drugs. However, the mechanisms of allogeneic rejection are different among the types of cells, tissues, and organs. Therefore, prevention and treatment strategies for allogeneic rejection are different.

This book includes nine chapters that provide recent evolutive information on scientific and therapeutic advances in allografting. In the section on solid organ allografts, chapters discuss prevention of rejection, pediatric ventricular assist devices, and desensitization. In the section on tissue allografts, chapters discuss success and ethical decision-making in vascularized composite allotransplantation, mitral valve allograft in the treatment of tricuspid valve pathology, the clinical implication of cardiac valve allografts in rare surgical circumstances, and allogeneic islet transplantation. In the section on particulate allografts, chapters discuss particulate allografts (DFDBA) combined with platelet concentrate for sinus lifts and post-extraction bone grafting in oral and maxillofacial surgery.

I would also like to thank all the contributors for their help in making this special book useful and interesting for readers.

Norihide Fukushima
Professor,
Senri Kinran University Graduate School of Nursing,
Suita, Japan

Visiting Director,
National Cerebral and Cardiovascular Center,
Suita, Japan

Section 1

Solid Organ Allograft

Chapter 1

Strategies for Prevention and Management of Heart Transplant Rejection

Estela Azeka

Abstract

Heart transplantation is the treatment of choice for patients with refractory heart failure treatment. Although there were advances in medical therapy and immunological knowledge regarding rejection, it is one of the major limitations for long-term survival for those who were submitted to heart transplantation. In this chapter, the main issues of rejection and prevention in heart transplantation will be discussed.

Keywords: heart transplantation, rejection, prevention, coronary vasculopathy, cellular rejection

1. Introduction

Heart transplantation has been the treatment of choice for patients with refractory heart failure or end-stage heart disease.

There are complications related to the heart transplant such as rejection, primary graft failure, cardiac allograft vasculopathy (CAV), and other complications due to the immunosuppressant drugs.

One of the major limitations to survival is still the rejection so prevention is the main challenge for those who take care of these patients after heart transplantation. In this chapter, the main issues of heart transplantation and prevention of rejection will be discussed.

The prevention of rejection starts when the recipient is evaluated for heart transplantation (pretransplant), during and after the procedure [1].

2. Pretransplant assessment protocol to establish personalized preventive strategies

2.1 Assessment of anti-HLA antibodies

Human leukocyte antigen (HLA) antibodies are important to detect because they are associated with rejection after transplantation.

Recently, the International Society of Heart and Lung Transplantation (ISHLT) published the updated Guidelines for the care of heart transplant recipients [2–5]. Most common antibody screening is performed by sensitive solid phase assay. Single antigen bead assays have allowed virtual crossmatching.

Antibody mean fluorescent intensity (MFI) is a method to assess the sensitization and help to determine a positive cross-match. It is a measure of antibody-antigen binding or HLA molecule bead saturation; however, it is affected by biological and technical factors.

The C1q assay is useful to identify antibodies capable of fixing complement. If C1q binds DSA strongly, this correlates with a positive cytotoxic crossmatch and it is associated with early antibody-mediated rejection.

The recommendation is: The anti-HLA class I and II specificities should be defined. In the absence of international standards, each center must define the antibody threshold for unacceptable risk. A mean MFI of less than 5000 is considered to be an acceptable threshold (Class I, Level of Evidence C) [2].

2.2 Panel reactive antibody (PRA) and risk factors for antibody-mediated rejection (AMR) or early phase acute rejection

The calculated panel reactive antibody (cPRA) is an estimation of the compatible donor pool collected when the recipient is evaluated for transplant and shows if the patient is sensitized or not. If the recipient has PRA > 10%, the patient is sensitized and has more risk to develop rejection after transplant as well as donor-directed antibodies [3].

There are some conditions where it is more common to have high PRA (**Table 1**).

It is important to monitor the cPRA because the serological presence of antibodies varies in the recipient over the time. For nonsensitized patients, HLA antibody screens are recommended every 6 months, and for sensitized patients every 3 months. For patients on mechanical assist support, after blood transfusions, infections, or using a desensitization therapy, HLA antibodies need to be evaluated every 1 to 2 weeks [2].

3. Desensitization methods: Brief protocols and outcome

The desensitization strategies are to decrease antibodies, B cells, plasma cells, and complement activation. There is no randomized clinical trial to assess the efficacy of the therapy. Furthermore, memory response may occur after antibody depletion. The protocols include perioperative plasmapheresis, IV immunoglobulin, or eculizumab at transplant [2].

Some centers have a protocol to desensitize these recipients using specific drugs and procedures (**Table 2**).

Previous surgery with pericardial bovine
Pregnancy
Previous transfusions

Table 1.
Conditions for sensitized patients.

Immunoglobulin
Rituximab
Plasmapheresis
Obinutuzumab
Bortezomib
Carfilzomib

Table 2.
Management for desensitization.

4. Donor-recipient matching and preventive way for hyperacute rejection or early phase antibody-mediated rejection

The recommendation for donor-recipient match at the time of transplant is a virtual crossmatch, which compares recipient anti-HLA antibody with donor HLA antigens (Class I, Level of Evidence C) [2].

Prospective or virtual crossmatch should be performed in recipient with PRA >10% (Class I, Level of Evidence C) [2].

Biopsies and circulating antibodies should be done routinely after transplantation. *De novo* donor-specific antibodies may be associated with poor outcome.

5. Preventive strategies after heart transplantation

The immunosuppressive regimen varies mainly according to the postoperative period and the diagnosis of type of rejection (**Table 3**). The rejection can be classified according to **Table 4** and graded according to pathologic findings.

The most common classification of immunosuppressive regimen is induction, maintenance, and treatment of rejection.

Endomyocardial biopsy remains the gold standard for the diagnosis of rejection. However, post-transplant rejection surveillance using endomyocardial biopsies has been decreasing over time due to the low number of positive biopsies in the era of calcineurin-inhibitor and mycophenolate-base immunosuppressive regimens.

So the emphasis is the use of noninvasive methods for surveillance of rejection, which has been increased. **Table 5** shows the main noninvasive methods for surveillance of rejection.

The immunosuppressive regimens are used to prevent rejection; however, it is difficult to balance between rejections and avoid the side effects of the drugs as well as infection and malignancy.

1. Induction therapy (early postoperative period)
2. Maintenance regimen (prevent rejection)
3. Treatment of rejection

Table 3.
Types of immunosuppressive regimens according to the posttransplant period.

Hyperacute rejection (humoral)
Acute rejection (cellular or humoral)
Chronic rejection (CAV coronary allograft vasculopathy)
Mixed rejection (cellular and humoral)

Table 4.
Types of rejection.

Biomarkers:
Cardiac troponins I and T
BNP
Assessment of immunologic risk predictors:
Genetic expression profiling
Donor-derived cell-free (DD cf-DNA)
Donor specific antibodies
Imaging methods
Chest ray
Echocardiogram
Cardiac MRI
ECG
Galium 67 scintigraphy

Table 5.
Noninvasive rejection monitoring.

Oyer et al. reported in 1983 the use of cyclosporine, as immunosuppressive drug for heart transplantation with improvement in survival. Since then, many regimens have been used to prevent rejection as well as renal insufficiency and posttransplant lymph proliferative diseases.

5.1 Induction therapy

The immune reactivity and the risk of rejection are high in the early postoperative period so the immunosuppressive regimens have the highest intensity after the procedure. This is one of the reasons that many centers use induction therapy and maintenance drugs with high target blood levels. Induction therapy is performed using antilymphocyte antibodies for specific epitopes on the surface of lymphocytes. The induction also allows delayed initiation of nephrotoxic drugs and weaning of glucocorticoid regimens.

The drugs that have been use for induction are interleukin-2 receptor antagonists and antilymphocyte antibodies (polyclonal antithymocyte antibodies and monoclonal antilymphocyte antibodies include alemtuzumab).

Interleukin-2 receptor antagonists are a monoclonal antibody that binds to the IL-2 receptor of T lymphocytes, blocking binding of IL-2 to the receptor complex so it inhibits IL-2-mediated T lymphocyte proliferation.

Polyclonal antilymphocyte antibodies act directly against human T-cell antigens. This causes a depletion of T lymphocytes.

According to the recent ISHLT update guidelines, induction with polyclonal antibody may be beneficial in patients with a high risk of renal dysfunction when used with intent to delay or avoid the use of a CNI (Class IIa, Level of Evidence B) [2].

In pediatric population, the use of IL-2 antagonist or polyclonal antibody induction is beneficial over corticosteroids (CS) only induction and is also recommended when CS-sparing or avoiding therapies are applied (Class II, Level of Evidence B) [2].

5.2 Standard maintenance immunosuppression, mechanism of action, indication, and outcome

The strategies of maintenance immunosuppression therapy have improved over time.

Calcineurin inhibitors (CNI), such as cyclosporine and tacrolimus, antimetabolite agent (azathioprine or mycophenolate), and glucocorticoids, are the most common combination of immunosuppressive protocols.

Proliferation signal inhibitors are used for renal insufficiency, cardiac allograft vasculopathy, and malignancy.

The updated guidelines of recipient care for ISHLT recommend:

1. Calcineurin inhibitor-based therapy remains the standard immunosuppressive protocol used after transplant (Class IIa, Level of Evidence B).

2. Mycophenolate, everolimus, and sirolimus should be included in contemporary immunosuppressive regimens because therapies, including these drugs, have been shown to reduce the onset and progression of CAV as assessed by IVUS (Class IIa. Level of Evidence B).

3. Sensitized recipients with evidence of donor-specific antibody (DSA) with high immunologic risk in pediatric recipients, tacrolimus is the preferred CNI (Class IIa, Level of Evidence C).

The most common maintenance immunosuppressive drugs are explained in **Table 6.**

Calcineurin inhibitors
Cyclosporin
Tacrolimus
Cytostatic drugs
Mycophenolate
Azathioprine
Steroids

Table 6.
Maintenance immunosuppressive drugs.

5.3 Surveilance of rejection

1. *Biomarkers* High-sensitivity cardiac troponins and BNP are useful to identify high-risk patients that need additional evaluation for ACR, AMR, or CAV (Class IIb, Level of Evidence C).

2. *Endomyocardial biopsy* is reasonable to be performed during the first 3 to 12 months after transplantation (Class IIa, Level of Evidence C).

3. *Echocardiogram* is acceptable as a rejection monitoring in patients at low risk for acute rejection and in whom EMB is not possible (Class IIb, Level of Evidence C).

4. *Posttransplant monitoring of DSA* should be performed at 1,3, 6, and 12 months and annually thereafter. Sensitized patients should be monitored more often (Class IIa, Level of Evidence C).

6. Classification of rejection

6.1 Classification of AMR

pAMR 0 negative for pathologic AMR: histopathologic and immunologic studies are both negatives [3, 6];

pAMR 1 (H+)—histopathologic AMR alone: histopathologic findings present and immunopathologic findings negative;

pAMR 1 (I+)—immunopathologic AMR alone: immunopathologic AMR alone: histopathologic findings negative and immunopathologic findings positive, that is, CD68+ and/or C4d + for IHC and C4d + with or without C3d + for IF.

pAMR 2—pathologic AMR: histopathologic and immunopathologic findings are both present.

pAMR 3 severe pathologic AMR: interstitial hemorrhage, capillary fragmentation, mixed inflammatory infiltrates, endothelial cell pyknosis, and/or karyorrhexis and marked edema and immunopathologic findings are present.

6.2 Classification of acute cellular rejection (ISHLT)

Grade 0—no rejection [7].

Grade 1R, mild—interstitial and/or perivascular infiltrate with up to one focus of myocyte damage.

Grade 2R, moderate—two or more foci of infiltrate with associated myocyte damage.

Grade 3R, severe—diffuse infiltrate with multifocal myocyte damage, with or without edema, hemorrhage, or vasculitis.

7. Rejection treatment

The treatment of rejection depends on the hemodynamic condition and the grading of rejection according to ISHLT grading. **Table 7** summarizes the therapeutic drugs

Grade II R or more and hemodynamic stable without vasoactive drugs:
Methylprednisolone
Grade II R or more and with vasoactive drugs
Methylprednisolone +Thymoglobulin + IVIG

Table 7.
Cellular rejection treatment.

in the rejection. Drugs for cellular rejection are *methylprednisolone, immunoglobulin (IVIG), rabbit thymoglobulin (ATG),* and maintenance immunosuppressive drugs [2].

The updated guidelines ISHLT recommends that patients with symptomatic acute cellular rejection should be hospitalized and patients with hemodynamic compromise should be treated in the ICU or an intermediate-care unit with the ability to perform continuous hemodynamic monitoring and administer inotropes (Class I, Level of Evidence C) [2].

The treatment for acute mediate rejection includes methylprednisolone, IVIG, ATG, rituximab, and plasmapheresis. In patients with severe rejection and not responsible for medical treatment, mechanical assistance support may be required.

8. Prevention for coronary allograft vasculopahy

One of the major limitations of heart transplantation is coronary allograft vasculopathy (CAV), which is called chronic rejection and occurs in 50% after 5 years of transplantation (**Figure 1**) [8–10]. The recommended nomenclature for cardiac allograft vasculopathy is based on the ISHLT proposed, adapted in **Table 8**. Coronary angiography is the gold standard for the diagnosis; however, in adult population, intravascular ultrasound can be used to detect coronary lesions as well as optical coherence tomography (OCT). **Table 9** shows the methods for CAV diagnosis.

Prevention for CAV includes some strategies described in **Table 10**.

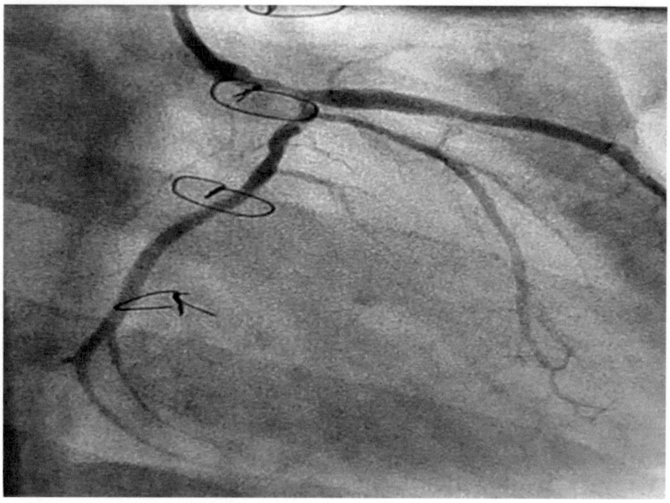

Figure 1.
Coronary angiography shows CAV lesions in left coronary artery.

ISHLT CAV 0 no detectable angiographic lesion
ISHLT CAV 1 mild
ISHLT CAV2 moderate
ISHLT CAV 3 severe

Table 8.
ISHLT CAV nomenclature (adapted).

Coronary angiography
Intravascular ultrasound (IVUS)
Optical coherence tomography (OCT)
Coronary computed tomographic angiography (CCTA)
Intracoronary flow (CFR, IMR)
PET myocardial blood flow quantification and perfusion imaging
DSE (dobutamine stress echocardiogram)

Table 9.
Methods for CAV diagnosis.

Control of cardiac risk factors (hypertension, diabetes, hyperlipidemia, smoking, obesity
Prevention CMV
Statin therapy
Substitution of mychophenolate or azathioprine to proliferation signal inhibitors

Table 10.
Prevention for CAV.

9. Conclusion

Prevention of rejection is one of the most important issues in heart transplantation. Although there are many drugs that can be used to prevent rejection, rejection is still one of the major complications after transplantation and causes of death.

Author details

Estela Azeka
Heart Institute (InCor) University of Sao Paulo Medical School, Sao Paulo, Brazil

*Address all correspondence to: estela_azeka9@hotmail.com

References

[1] Daly K. Contemporary transplantation immunosuppression: Balancing on the immunosuppression seesaw. In: Canter C, Everitt E, Burch M, Louis JD, editors. Pediatric Heart Transplantation. Kirklin KJ, series editor. ISHLT Monograph Series. Chicago, IL: ISHLT; 2019. pp. 52-93

[2] Velleca A, Shullo MA, Dhital K, et al. The International Society for Heart and Lung Transplantation (ISHLT) guidelines for the care of heart transplant recipients. The Journal of Heart and Lung Transplantation. 2023;**42**(5):e1-e141

[3] Colvin MM, Cook JL, Chang PM et al. Antibody-mediated rejection in cardiac transplantation: Emerging knowledge in diagnosis and management a scientific statement from the American Heart Association. Circulation. 2015;**131**(18):1608-1639. Available from: http://circ.ahajournals.org/

[4] Rao RA, Kransdorf EP, Patel JK, et al. How to approach HLA sensitization in heart transplant candidates. JACC: Heart Failure. 2023;**11**(4):469-475

[5] Lefaucheur C, Louis K, Morris AB, STAR 2022 Working Group, et al. Clinical recommendations for posttransplant assessment of anti-HLA (human leukocyte antigen) donor-specific antibodies: A sensitization in transplantation: Assessment of risk consensus document. American Journal of Transplantation. 2023;**23**(1):115-132

[6] Berry GJ, Burke M, Andersen C, et al. The 2013 International Society for Heart and Lung Transplantation working formulation for the standardization of nomenclature in the pathologic diagnosis of antibody-mediated rejection in heart transplantation. The Journal of Heart and Lung Transplantation. 2013;**32**(12):1147-1162

[7] Stewart S, Winters GL, Fishbein MC, et al. ISHLT consensus report. Revision of the 1990 working formulation for the standardization of nomenclature in the diagnosis of heart rejection. The Journal of Heart and Lung Transplantation. 2005;**24**:1710-1720

[8] Spartalis M, Spartalis E, Tzatzaki E, et al. Cardiac allograft vasculopathy after heart transplantation: Current prevention and treatment strategies. European Review for Medical and Pharmacological Sciences. 2019;**23**(1):303-311

[9] Mehra MR. Contemporary concepts in prevention and treatment of cardiac allograft vasculopathy. American Journal of Transplantation. 2006;**6**(6):1248-1256

[10] Mehra MR, Crespo-Leiro MG, Dipchand A, et al. International Society for Heart and Lung Transplantation working formulation of standardized nomenclature for cardiac allograft vasculopathy-2010. The Journal of Heart and Lung Transplantation. 2010;**29**(38):1056-1066

Chapter 2

Pediatric Ventricular Assist Devices

Madonna Lee

Abstract

In the past 2 decades, pediatric mechanical circulatory support (MCS) strategies have improved. Focus on ventricular assist devices (VAD) is an important topic for pediatric heart failure patients and single ventricle palliation. Application of VADs continues to evolve, including implanting compact adult continuous-flow devices to larger children (HeartMate 3) along with the recent discontinuation of the HeartWare. The Berlin Heart ExCOR has received improved outcomes with adjustments to anticoagulation. Syncardia Total Artificial Heart has also released a smaller version which has been implanted in adolescents. Advanced cross-sectional imaging can now be used for pre-operative planning of device placement. Finally, special consideration is required for usage of these devices in a failing Fontan circulation (univentricular physiology) with some lab studies and small cases highlighting the unique challenges. The potential options for VAD as a bridge to transplant, destination therapy, or recovery continue to expand the crucial role of MCS in congenital heart disease. Smaller patient size, limited availability of organs for heart transplant, and longer survival of pediatric congenital patients continues to make innovation in MCS necessary.

Keywords: children heart failure, mechanical circulatory support, congenital, single ventricle, ventricular assist devices, anticoagulation

1. Introduction

For patients with severe end-stage heart failure, there are limited therapeutic options past medical goal-directed therapy. The surgical options for treatment of pediatric congenital patients who require mechanical circulatory support (MCS) is gradually increasing with many opportunities for ongoing research, clinical studies, and device innovation. This chapter will focus specifically on ventricular assist devices (VAD) in a pediatric population. Subtopics will include research within the past few decades, size and availability of pediatric devices, anticoagulation, and special anatomic considerations in congenital heart disease (CHD).

2. Sizing and device selection

One of the biggest challenges in utilizing MCS devices in young children is the limited availability of products for a range of patients that are not yet adult-sized. There are several ways to combat this in order to find the optimal available device. One is to identify the currently available range of devices for use in pediatrics. With technological advances in imaging, pre-operative digital modeling can help with preoperative planning. And, lastly, there are currently trials for more products that will hopefully become available for use in children to increase the availability of MCS devices.

2.1 Preoperative advanced imaging and three-dimensional printing

One of the advantages of utilization advanced imaging and customizable technology in congenital heart disease patients is the ability to adapt to variable anatomy. Surgical aspects of implanting a device may benefit from newer technologies such as preoperative computed tomography (CT) or three-dimensional (3D) printing. A few examples include cannula placement and device location in adults with congenital heart disease and heart failure.

Recent usage of this technology over the past two decades requires specific resources including excellent dataset image acquisition, image processing software, a variety of printing materials, and a 3D printer [1]. In Ref. [1], usage in various adult cardiac and congenital heart patients is explored demonstrating interest with multiple clinically useful applications including patient/family education, training, and operative planning. Some interesting case examples include VAD implantation in a failing systemic right ventricle or after Fontan palliation [2]. In Ref. [3], multiple 3D printed models are shown including color cardiac models and a whole-chest with sternum/ribs along with other soft tissue to simulate the ideal location of a VAD device for a congenital heart patient. The future of 3D printing and MCS offers a unique ability to personalize each patient's anatomy. Although an exciting new tool, the barriers to increased adoption of this technology include cost, inability to print certain valve structures, access to software, image datasets acquisition expertise, printing materials that closely replicate living tissue, personnel, and 3D printers [1, 2].

In terms of precise preoperative management and placement of VADs, the ability to acquire and measure using CT imaging offers an advantage, especially when assessing children who may be borderline candidates due to smaller thoracic cavity size. Some anthropometric measures include chest cavity dimensions (i.e. internal transverse diameter at different levels, etc.). Patients as young as 8 years-old have been described as receiving implantation, with others from 9 to 11 years of age undergoing preoperative CT imaging and successful implantation. One of the major obstacles to placing a sparse selection of VAD device sizes is compromising the position of the pump after closing the chest. Due to patient size variability, CT imaging offers an objective measure to determine feasibility and evaluate technical implantation preoperatively [4].

2.2 Available implantable devices

Currently, out of over 200 annual pediatric device implantations worldwide, there are only a few types of devices that are available for use in pediatric patients [5]. Another additive factor includes an increase in heart failure hospitalizations in the pediatric population requiring increased usage of these devices, specifically for CHD [5, 6]. There are two broad categories of VAD implantable devices: continuous-flow and pulsatile. The majority of devices being implanted since 2014 are continuous-flow due to the miniaturization and availability of these adult intracorporeal devices to be placed into adolescents [7]. One of the devices which was available for implantation was recently recalled due to thrombosis risk: Heartware (Medtronic, MN, US) [4]. In a 2019 published article [8], the database of the Pediatric Interagency Registry for

Mechanical Circulatory Support (Pedimacs), reviewed recent outcomes for children with VADs. There were 108 CHD patients over about 5-year span and these were compared to non-CHD patients; CHD patients tended to be younger and smaller (average age 5.7 years with BSA 0.8 m^2) [8]. This study found that CHD was associated with an increased mortality and decreased transplant rates; however, the subgroup who received implantable devices at high volume centers had higher survival rates [8]. There is a consistent trend with increased numbers of children being implanted with these devices within the last decade [5]. Although limited, clinical trials are on-going to make smaller and improved devices for use in pediatrics.

2.2.1 Berlin Heart EXCOR

A pulsatile, paracorporeal ventricular assist device currently approved for pediatric use is the Berlin Heart EXCOR (Berlin Heart, Inc., The Woodlands, TX, US) [9]. Since the first implantation in 1990s, this device offers multiple pump sizes ranging from 10 to 80 mL stroke volume to be assigned based on the patient's body surface area (BSA) [10]. In Ref. [10], comparison of 80 patients divided into three groups with an optimally sized pump matching stroke volume to BSA, it appeared that thrombotic events were more frequent statistically significantly in children who had a larger pump placed in comparison to BSA. Also, in a much smaller patient (i.e. <3 kg), the smallest pump (10 mL) may need to be run at a rate that is much lower than the optimal heart rate resulting in lower flow and potentially a risk for thrombosis [9]. One potential solution is to insert an assist device on the right and left ventricular in order to maintain a high enough output [9]. There are studies showing some decrease in survival with biventricular support; however, this may be due to the advanced stages of heart failure, which may be alleviated with earlier implementation of univentricular support [10]. Also, patients less than 5 kg were disproportionately at risk for death, possibly due to size mismatch of the device compared to intrinsic native cardiac output in small infants [9]. There are good results for ultimate transplantation or even recovery; however, there is also noted a high incidence of bleeding and thrombosis. Reference [10] studied a total of 80 children who underwent Berlin Heart implantation. They found that 25 children died (mortality rate of 31.6%); 49% of patients were successfully transplanted and 19% of devices explanted. BSA, young age, or having biventricular support did not appear to be associated with increased mortality – potentially attributable to increased experience. Other technical aspects such as site of cannulation or coated cannulas may also lead to improved results [10]. Another limitation of this device is training of hospital personnel and requirements of staying inpatient for device monitoring.

2.2.2 HeartMate 3

The HeartMate 2 and HeartMate 3 (Abbott, Abbott Park, IL, US) are two devices that are implantable compact continuous-flow VADs designed for use in adults that is being implanted in children [9]. However, the HeartMate 2 is no longer the preferred device in this age group. Some older studies, such as reference [9], authors describe their experience at their institution of developing education and support so that there is comfort and experience in implanting HeartMate 2 devices and allowing pediatric patients to be discharged home and managed as an outpatient. This was a significant improvement from the paracorporeal or centrifugal devices requiring management in the hospital. The MOMENTUM 3 trial released the results for usage of the HeartMate

3 which can provide flows between 2.5 L/min and 10 L/min and alternating rotor speeds every other second [9].

The recall of the other lower profile device, discussed in the subsequent section, has made implementation of HeartMate 3 as the ideal device for smaller patients, with an outer diameter of 50 mm [4]. In [11] the early experience described by the Advanced Cardiac Therapies Improving Outcomes Network (ACTION) published in 2020, 35 patients from 2017 to 2019 at multiple centers had a HeartMate 3 implanted in pediatric and adult patients with congenital heart disease. There were patients as small as 19 kg who were successfully implanted and supported (median age = 15.7) – establishing this device as a feasible option for adolescents [11]. Currently, the consensus for appropriate device usage is for older children or young adults weighing greater than 30 kg, although there is no minimum weight restriction [5]. Research is on-going regarding utilization of preoperative advanced imaging to virtually plan implantation.

2.2.3 HeartWare HVAD

The HeartWare HVAD (HeartWare, Inc., Framingham, MA, US) is another implantable compact continuous-flow VAD that was designed for adults and was being implanted in older children [9]. As in Ref. [9], as of recently, there were excitement and documented case reports describing successful implantation of this compact option even in a child as small as 13 kg and as young as 4 years old for over 600 days. There were published studies from a multicenter study describing the implantation in small children. They described a 33% rate of pump thrombosis yet at this single center, Burki et al. describe no pump thrombosis out of 19 patients [9]. However, this device was discontinued after the rates of thrombosis were very high. Unfortunately, it is no longer an option. Without this device as an option, it is difficult to know what the smaller threshold would have been to avoid patient-device size mistmatch between very small children and adult-designed VADs [9].

Over 5 years, it appeared that the implantation of HVAD was steadily increasing through 2017. Even worldwide, there was reported success in children in achieving goal to transplant – over 200 patients from 2015 to 2016 [12]. Perhaps, this was from the innovation of implantation techniques, and even reports demonstrating improvement with biventricular support. Unfortunately, despite these successes, in 2021, the Heartware HVAD was withdrawn completely from the market. Overall, this was a huge setback for the field, but since this was one of two smaller profile devices that were most commonly used in pediatrics, there is currently a gap in comparison to experience versus now this device being unavailable for implantation. HeartMate 3 devices may be able to address the gap for patients that are greater than 30 kg with an adequate chest cavity size. However, practically, given the prevalence of the Berlin Heart as being the only other device having available device sizes from 15 to 30 kg, the removal of the HVAD from markets leaves yet another gap for smaller children less than 30 kg. This is not an ideal replacement, since the Berlin Heart currently requires an inpatient admission without the ability for patients to be discharged home [5]. The impact of this recent device disappearing from the already limited toolkit of the pediatric cardiac surgeon is estimated to have a significant clinical impact without an immediate solution.

2.2.4 Other devices

The Syncardia Total Artificial Heart (Syncardia, Inc., Tuscon, AZ, US) is an option with size constraints to the pumps: a smaller pump 50 mL for the pediatric population which was made available in 2022 and the pre-existing 70 mL pump which is too large for most pediatric patients [9].

Short-term, centrifugal paracorporeal devices using in smaller children such as the PediMag, RotaFlow, or CentriMag (Abbott, Abbott Park, IL, US) are all important as contemporary options for mechanical circulatory support for inpatients who are critically ill [5]. However, the discussion of the usage of these devices compared to implantable durable devices is beyond the scope of this chapter.

2.3 Device development

Currently, there very few clinical trials with device development geared specifically towards pediatric patients [5]. Unfortunately, progress has been slow and halting. Resources are limited. Reasons studies are lacking and difficulty in making substantial progress with a potentially life-saving device are multifactorial including small consumer numbers, substantial regulatory and administrative burden, and patient variability [9]. One potential solution is to encourage device development for both adults and pediatrics [5]. The MVAD (Heartware, Inc.) is another adult-size continuous-flow compact device undergoing testing with a volume of 20 mL [9]. Despite multiple studies originally being funded, there is only one that is currently on-going specifically for pediatrics [7]. The most well-described, smallest device is the Jarvik Infant 2015 which is a continuous-flow VAD targeted towards children 8 kg to 20 kg; the device length is about equal to a AA-battery [9, 13]. The difficulty in performing research in this specific area has been well-described by the lead investigators at Texas Heart Institute [7, 13]. One of the biggest hurtles in developing this device was addressing hemolysis [9]. Another obstacle is the concern for thrombosis. This comes from the inherent patient-device mismatch from implanting adult devices into pediatric patients [7]. Finally, this long awaited device specifically designed for kids will be ready to enroll patients in the PumpKIN (pumps for kids, infants, and neonates) trial [7, 9, 13]. We eagerly await the results for at least another feasible option in the treatment of young children.

3. Anticoagulation

One of the biggest challenges in children and MCS is achieving the ideal balance between bleeding and anticoagulation to prevent thrombosis. This balance is particularly difficult to achieve in pediatric patients due to alterations in hemostasis during development, pro-inflammatory states, or various genetic syndromes [9]. Pharmocologic regimens and combinations differ with a variety of options including the usage of a heparin infusion, low-molecular-weight-heparin, anti-platelet therapy, direct thrombin inhibitors, or warfarin. In addition to differences in pharmacology, target goals and measurements for monitoring are also variable. In the Berlin EXCOR study evaluating pump size [10], this institution describes measuring anti-Xa levels, international normalized ratio, as well as obtaining thromboelastography and platelet aggregation tests for patients also being treated with acetylsalicyclic acid and dipyridamole (or clopidogrel) to ensure therapeutic effect. Reported thrombosis rates for the Berlin Heart are 20–29%. It is hypothesized that larger pump size, due to limitations of appropriate device size for patient body, may be a risk for thromboembolic events [10]. There is variability in whether studies find that <10 kg body weight is a risk factor for thrombosis. Optimal protocols and regimes have been studied to decrease the risk of thromboembolic events while also keeping rates of bleeding low, especially around the perioperative period.

4. Clinical pathways after device implantation

There are several clinical outcomes for children after VAD implantation. It seems that there are increased hospitalizations for decompensated heart failure and more utilization of VADs. Mechanical circulatory device clinical pathways can include bridge-to-transplant, bridge-to-recovery, or currently alive [6]. If it is unknown whether the patient will be suitable for transplant, bridge-to-decision is also an option, but less likely for a durable device in the era of other temporary MCS options. A subset of patients may also require biventricular assist device placement in both the right and left ventricle. Given the growing number of device implantation in children, it is imperative that we continue to review early and late outcomes, as well as measure the impact of quality of life (QOL) in these complex patients.

4.1 Bridge-to-transplant

Some CHD patients may fail surgical repair or multi-stage surgical palliation and require bridging support prior to heart transplantation. One of the benefits of implanting durable VADs in children awaiting transplant is the improved posttransplant survival and decreased waitlist times compared to using temporary mechanical circulatory support such as ECMO. This includes improved nutrition, function of other organs, and rehab prior to transplant – with reports of increased VAD utilization in this pediatric population. Unfortunately, the number of pediatric heart transplantation donors continues to be static within North America [5].

In the most recent era, reference [14] studied the pediatric VAD implantation across two eras (1999 to 2004 or 2005 to 2012). There have been more pediatric patients listed Status 1A – indicating the highest critical need. However, despite this increase, there has been a significant decrease from 2005 to 2012 of 50% in transplant waitlist mortality compared to the previous era. Risk factors for waitlist mortality included weight < 10 kg, CHD, ECMO, mechanical ventilation, or renal dysfunction. VAD was protective and improved waitlist survival [14].

When analyzing whether racial disparities exist in post-transplant survival after VAD implantation, reference [15] elucidates that disparities still exist. Studies have shown that racial minorities experience inferior outcomes after heart transplant. Black children were most ill with a greater proportion Status 1A. Outcomes at 1-year post-transplant were equivalent, but long-term survival was worse for non-whites. On multivariable analysis, black race independently predicted mortality. This study showed that even though the most ill patients receive VADs, with similar pretransplant and early transplant outcomes, black and Hispanic pediatric patients experienced inferior post-transplant survival after VAD as a bridge-to-transplant.

4.2 Biventricular assist device support

Another portion of CHD patients after placement of left VAD may experience severe right ventricular dysfunction, necessitating a right VAD: biventricular assist device (BiVAD) support. In adults, attempts have been made to identify risk factors and subsequent risk scoring to try and predict which patients may need both ventricles supported [16, 17]. Physiologically, LVAD support may augment worsening RVAD failure through many factors, but predicting the level to which a second device placement is warranted is difficult [18]. In Ref. [18], authors reviewed long-term VAD implantation to try and identify risk factors. Unfortunately, patients requiring temporary right VAD support or BiVAD support were at increased risk of mortality [12, 18]. Also, emergent RVAD implantation was associated with worse outcomes. After multivariate logistic regression indicated that decreased milrinone application was a preoperative risk factor associated with requiring BiVAD instead of sole left VAD support. But, in other terms, patients who received preoperative milrinone had decreased odds of developing right heart dysfunction, which was statistically significant [18]. This paralleled some findings in adults as well [17]. However, none of the many other variables evaluated were correlated with predisposing to BiVAD support. It was also observed that the frequency of BiVAD placement in pediatric patients has been decreasing, possibly from improved implantation techniques [18].

4.3 Outcomes and quality of life

In the past few decades, outcomes for pediatric VAD implantation continue to improve. Patients can be successfully bridged to transplant in over 20% of patients [19]. Unfortunately, some of the outcomes data are currently outdated due to use in previous studies of devices that are no longer available [9, 12]. In the early experience of HeartMate 3, short-term follow-up of 35 patients demonstrated an early survival of 97%, with only one mortality [11]. Almost 60% were able to achieve transplantation. Early results were encouraging with no stroke or pump thrombosis after an average of 3-months of follow-up. Not evaluating just by device type, the larger registry among the 471 patients enrolled in the Pediatric Interagency Registry for Mechanical Circulatory Support from 2012 until 2017, groups were divided looking at outcomes for biventricular versus single ventricle patients, specifically with CHD, compared with non-CHD pediatric patients [8]. At 6 months, CHD patients had a higher mortality (36.4%) compared to non-CHD VAD patients (12.1%) and almost half transplantation rate of 29% versus 60%. However, this study also included patients with paracorporeal devices as well as implantable continuous devices. Despite looking at multiple variables, CHD seemed to be the highest association of mortality with VAD placement. As experience with implantation and increased number of children receiving these devices, more data from large registries will be able to help predict which patients will achieve the best outcomes from VAD implantation [9].

One of the earliest studies to compare outcomes of Berlin Heart to ECMO for bridge to transplant demonstrated that longer duration of support without significant risk of stroke and suggested improved survival on Berlin versus ECMO: 86% versus 56%. An updated study looking at more children in 47 centers identified about 200 children requiring support between 2007 and 2010, with median duration of support 40 days. The authors concluded that with the dramatic rise in usage, about 75% of patients survived to transplant or recovery. Risk factors associated with mortality included smaller patients, renal/hepatic dysfunction, and use of biventricular support [20].

Another large, single-center summarized the morbidity for patients requiring MCS associated with mortality from 1998 to 2007. In [21], some major complications the authors noted included infection, respiratory failure, major bleeding, hepatic/renal failure, right heart failure, and neurologic injury. They cited major neurologic injury occurring in almost half of the 25 patients. Although survival to transplant was still three-quarters, consistent with other reports, the monitoring of neuro status changes continues to be challenging requiring aggressive evaluation for potential injury with patient sympatoms.

In a prospective study from 2014, VAD questionnaires were administered to parents to assess children's Pediatric Quality of Life Inventory pre- and post- VAD placement [19]. These scores were compared to healthy children, outpatients with heart failure, and children after heart transplant. Out of 13 patients, 11 were able to receive a heart transplant and one was still alive on VAD support. Patients reported lower physical QOL scores and lower psychosocial scores. In Ref. [22], 82 children from the Pediatric Interagency Registry for Mechanical Circulatory Support completed a self-report quality of life assessment from pre- and post- VAD implantation. QOL scores were lower than normal for physical and psychosocial scores in both groups pre-VAD. However, it appeared that psychosocial scores improved in children post-VAD at 3 and 6 months post-op. Patients seemed to be mostly concerned physically with being unable to resume usual play activities compared to other children. However, this survey suggests that VAD placement may improve children's psychosocial health after implantation.

5. Special anatomic congenital considerations

Another challenge in utilizing MCS devices in children or adults with congenital heart disease is the incredible amount of variation that occurs either at birth or after multiple palliative operations. We discuss some of these specific examples to highlight the challenges and the limited data available on current usage. Although this appears to be increasing, the practical application of MCS to these challenging patient cases will require more experience and long-term follow-up.

5.1 Single ventricle patients

Single ventricle patients who undergo staged palliation requiring partial or complete cavopulmonary anastomosis present a unique challenge to implementation of MCS. These challenges include technical/anatomic differences in these patients, as well as physiologic. However, this population is also at significant risk for heart failure during the interstages between Stage I (Norwood or Hybrid), Stage II (bidirectional Glenn), and Stage III (Fontan operation). For example, the authors from Kansas City describe a case report supplying MCS in a superior cavopulmonary patient as a bridge to transplant in an infant [23]. In **Figure 1** [23], the authors illustrate cannulation in the reconstructed aortic root (Damus-Kaye-Stansel) and systemic ventricle for a failing Glenn patient. They describe the patient's changes in physiology while maintained on support and prior to successful transplantation after one year. They conclude that successful long-term support is feasible and ECMO in parallel can be instituted as a strategy for short-term pulmonary support [23].

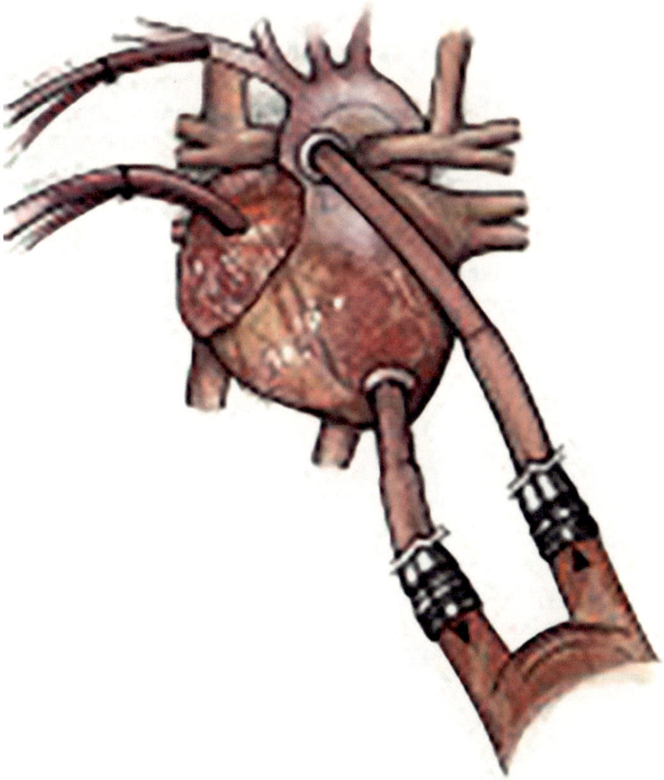

Figure 1.
Ref. [23]. Reprinted with permission from Elsevier under CC-BY-ND-ND license.

The Fontan operation is typically the final staged palliation for single ventricle patients that connects the systemic venous return to the pulmonary circulation (total cavopulmonary anastomosis). In Ref. [24], a broad description of the background, physiology, and details of different types of Fontan surgically created circulation can be reviewed for building a knowledge foundation. The failing Fontan is another category of research that elucidates the inherent challenge in these patients of ultimately needing a heart transplant [25]. This patient population can be particularly medically challenging due to manifestations of chronic Fontan circulation including liver dysfunction, valve regurgitation, myocardial dysfunction, collaterals, plastic bronchitis, and protein-losing enteropathy. With the addition of anatomic and physiologic challenges, inserting MCS devices into this population is currently under review. Fontan failure can be multifactorial with cardiovascular factors including ventricular dysfunction [6]. Once failure symptomatology starts, transplant waitlist mortality is high [6]. Several limited options exist for supporting failing Fontan physiology including VAD implantation [6, 26].

Using VADs addresses myocardial failure, but will not reverse cavopulmonary failure. Currently, there are no pumps specifically designed for Fontan cavopulmonary circulation. Implantation of these devices may be anatomically challenging due to prevalent under development of one ventricle – leading patients down a single-ventricle pathway. Despite these challenges, some bench research has supported using of the VAD successfully in failing Fontan circulation. Also, the HeartMate 2 supported a sheep for 2 hours when placed in the cavopulmonary graft. Implantation of the HeartWare HVAD in three Fontan patients for 5 to 9 months were successful bridge to transplant [26]. However, in 2021, the HeartWare device was recalled and not currently available for implantation [5]. One case demonstrated the Berlin Heart provided biventricular support for a failing Fontan circulation [26]. HeartMate 3 implantation in a CHD Fontan patient is usually performed after multiple previous staged palliative operations [6].

One of the physiologic challenges after insertion of VAD into the ventricle is off-loading, but can also concomitantly increase Fontan pressures, which can lead to a worsening clinical situation. It does appear that continuous devices are more beneficial than pulsatile devices given the reliance of the circulation on passive pulmonary flow [26]. Careful consideration is needed of the underlying etiology for a failing Fontan, such as ventricular failure, elevated pulmonary artery pressures, or end-diastolic pressures.

In Ref. [6], the Society of Thoracic Surgeons created a group dedicated to observing the outcomes of Fontan patients supported with VADs from 2012 to 2019 using large mechanical assist device registries (Pedimacs and Intermacs). Retrospectively, they found 55 Fontan patients with a median age of 10 years and 27 kg who underwent VAD implantation. Highlighting the trend of more device implantation and growing experience, the equivalent number of VADs were implanted in the last year of observation compared to the previous 5 years (28 vs. 27; $p = 0.01$, from 2018 to 2019 and 2012–2017, respectively). In addition, the later era had a higher pre-VAD glomerular filtration rate, perhaps demonstrating earlier implantation. Overwhelmingly (89%) of devices were placed to support the systemic ventricle as left-sided VADs. The overall positive outcome (alive, transplant, or recovery) was demonstrated in 81% at 6 months with median length of support at 3.8 months. Fifty-eight percent of all mortality occurred during the first month. Demonstrating the length of duration VAD support can offer, five patients received support for greater than 1 year. Adverse events such as stroke, pump thrombosis, and bleeding ranged from 4 to 9% (1.4 to 3.3 out of 100 patient-months). Important implantation considerations in Fontan patients includes perioperative care, aortopulmonary collaterals, pulmonary vascular disease, or end organ dysfunction can coexist [6].

5.2 Surgical modifications

Currently, some alternative surgical techniques to implanting devices through a median sternotomy and placing the device intrapericardially are under investigation. A minimally invasive approach using two anterior thoracotomies or hemisternotomy are being explored with multiple potential advantages. Because it may be difficult to align the inflow cannula vertically, so that it lies parallel to the interventricular septum, another implantation technique is to divide the left hemidiaphragm to create a pump pocket, as described by reference [9]. Surgical modifications of tunneling the driveline in under-developed abdominal walls of smaller children may decrease an already elevated risk of driveline infections in this population by off-setting the insertion through the rectus abdominis muscle [9]. Resecting papillary muscle that may cause mechanical obstruction, reorienting the direction of the outflow, and padding the pump housing against the chest to try and decrease pain with a buffer are other surgical techniques described when treating smaller congenital heart disease patients [4].

6. Conclusions

With recent device innovations, there are more options than ever before for pediatric congenital heart disease patients. However, special considerations still need to be given to specific congenital anomalies and patients with single ventricles. Risks of anticoagulation with bleeding and thrombosis are also careful considerations. There has been tremendous progress in the realm of MCS for pediatric patients in end-stage heart failure, but more research focusing on device and pharmacologic improvements needs to be done.

Conflict of interest

The author declares no conflict of interest.

Author details

Madonna Lee
Division of Cardiac Surgery, Department of Surgery, Yale School of Medicine, New Haven, Connecticut, USA

*Address all correspondence to: madonna.lee@yale.edu

References

[1] Henn MC, Mokadam NA. Three-dimensional printing to plan intracardiac operations. JTCVS Techniques. 2021;**9**:101-108

[2] Farooqi KM, Saeed O, Zaidi A, Sanz J, Nielsen JC, Hsu DT, et al. 3D printing to guide ventricular assist device placement in adults with congenital heart disease and heart failure. JACC Heart Failure. 2016;**4**(4):301-311

[3] Miller JR, Singh GK, Woodard PK, Eghtesady P, Anwar S. 3D printing for preoperative planning and surgical simulation of ventricular assist device implantation in a failing systemic right ventricle. Journal of Cardiovascular Computed Tomography. 2020;**14**(6):e172-e1e4

[4] Van Puyvelde J, Jacobs S, Vlasselaers D, Meyns B. Heartmate 3 implantation in small patients: CT-guided chest diameter assessment. Interactive Cardiovascular and Thoracic Surgery. 2022;**34**(5):939-940

[5] Deshpande SR, Slepian MJ, Alsoufi B. HeartWare HVAD market withdrawal and impact on the Pediatric field. ASAIO Journal. 2021;**67**(8):825-826

[6] Bedzra EKS, Adachi I, Peng DM, Amdani S, Jacobs JP, Koehl D, et al. Systemic ventricular assist device support of the Fontan circulation yields promising outcomes: An analysis of the Society of Thoracic Surgeons Pedimacs and Intermacs databases. The Journal of Thoracic and Cardiovascular Surgery. 2022;**164**(2):353-364

[7] Adachi I. Current status and future perspectives of the PumpKIN trial. Translational Pediatrics. 2018;**7**(2):162-168

[8] Peng DM, Koehl DA, Cantor RS, McMillan KN, Barnes AP, McConnell PI, et al. Outcomes of children with congenital heart disease implanted with ventricular assist devices: An analysis of the Pediatric interagency registry for mechanical circulatory support (Pedimacs). The Journal of Heart and Lung Transplantation. 2019;**38**(4):420-430

[9] Burki S, Adachi I. Pediatric ventricular assist devices: Current challenges and future prospects. Vascular Health and Risk Management. 2017;**13**:177-185

[10] Miera O, Schmitt KRL, Delmo-Walter E, Ovroutski S, Hetzer R, Berger F. Pump size of Berlin heart EXCOR pediatric device influences clinical outcome in children. The Journal of Heart and Lung Transplantation. 2014;**33**(8):816-821

[11] O'Connor MJ, Lorts A, Davies RR, Fynn-Thompson F, Joong A, Maeda K, et al. Early experience with the HeartMate 3 continuous-flow ventricular assist device in pediatric patients and patients with congenital heart disease: A multicenter registry analysis. The Journal of Heart and Lung Transplantation. 2020;**39**(6):573-579

[12] Conway J, Miera O, Adachi I, Maeda K, Eghtesady P, Henderson HT, et al. Worldwide experience of a durable centrifugal flow pump in Pediatric patients. Seminars in Thoracic and Cardiovascular Surgery. 2018;**30**(3): 327-335

[13] Baldwin JT, Adachi I, Teal J, Almond CA, Jaquiss RD, Massicotte MP, et al. Closing in on the PumpKIN trial of the Jarvik 2015 ventricular assist device. Seminars in Thoracic and Cardiovascular

Surgery. Pediatric Cardiac Surgery Annual. 2017;**20**:9-15

[14] Zafar F, Castleberry C, Khan MS, Mehta V, Bryant R, Lorts A, et al. Pediatric heart transplant waiting list mortality in the era of ventricular assist devices. The Journal of Heart and Lung Transplantation. 2015;**34**(1):82-88

[15] Greenberg JW, Bryant R, Villa C, Fields K, Fynn-Thompson F, Zafar F, et al. Racial disparity exists in the utilization and post-transplant survival benefit of ventricular assist device support in children. The Journal of Heart and Lung Transplantation. 2023;**42**(5):585-592

[16] Fitzpatrick JR 3rd, Frederick JR, Hsu VM, Kozin ED, O'Hara ML, Howell E, et al. Risk score derived from pre-operative data analysis predicts the need for biventricular mechanical circulatory support. The Journal of Heart and Lung Transplantation. 2008;**27**(12):1286-1292

[17] Matthews JC, Koelling TM, Pagani FD, Aaronson KD. The right ventricular failure risk score a pre-operative tool for assessing the risk of right ventricular failure in left ventricular assist device candidates. Journal of the American College of Cardiology. 2008;**51**(22):2163-2172

[18] Fan Y, Zhang AM, Weng YG, Huebler M, Miera O, Franz N, et al. Factors associated with the need of biventricular mechanical circulatory support in children with advanced heart failure. European Journal of Cardio-Thoracic Surgery. 2013;**43**(5):1028-1035

[19] Miller JR, Boston US, Epstein DJ, Henn MC, Lawrance CP, Kallenbach J, et al. Pediatric quality of life while supported with a ventricular assist device. Congenital Heart Disease. 2015;**10**(4):E189-E196

[20] Almond CS, Morales DL, Blackstone EH, Turrentine MW, Imamura M, Massicotte MP, et al. Berlin heart EXCOR pediatric ventricular assist device for bridge to heart transplantation in US children. Circulation. 2013;**127**(16):1702-1711

[21] Stein ML, Robbins R, Sabati AA, Reinhartz O, Chin C, Liu E, et al. Interagency registry for mechanically assisted circulatory support (INTERMACS)-defined morbidity and mortality associated with pediatric ventricular assist device support at a single US center: The Stanford experience. Circulation. Heart Failure. 2010;**3**(6):682-688

[22] Peng DM, Yu S, Lowery R, Ventresco C, Cousino MK, St Louis JD, et al. Self-reported quality of life in children with ventricular assist devices. Pediatric Transplantation. 2022;**26**(4):e14237

[23] Bedzra EKS, Barnes A, Birnbaum B, St Louis JD. Mechanical support of superior cavopulmonary (Glenn) physiology to heart transplantation. JTCVS Techniques. 2021;**6**:144-146

[24] Lee M, Shahjehan RD. Fontan Completion. StatPearls. Treasure Island (FL): StatPearls Publishing; 2023. Available from: https://www.ncbi.nlm.nih.gov/books/NBK558950/

[25] Goldberg DJ, Shaddy RE, Ravishankar C, Rychik J. The failing Fontan: Etiology, diagnosis and management. Expert Review of Cardiovascular Therapy. 2011;**9**(6):785-793

[26] Zwischenberger JB, Breetz KA, Ballard-Croft C, Wang D. Failing Fontan cardiovascular support: Review. Journal of Cardiac Surgery. 2022;**37**(12):5257-5261

Chapter 3

Desensitization in Solid Organ Transplantation

Asad Ullah and Khalid AlMeshari

Abstract

Solid organ transplantation (SOT) has revolutionized the management of end-stage organ disease. Human Leukocyte antigen (HLA) sensitization and ABO incompatibility (ABOi) pose formidable barrier to SOT. The risk of acute rejection is high. They wait longer for compatible organs than their counterparts do. Furthermore, the graft and patient survival are suboptimal in incompatible transplants. Access to SOT could be promoted in this population by prioritizing them to well-matched organs in the allocation system *via* acceptable mismatch or paired donation programs. If these strategies fail to achieve transplantation, desensitization could provide an alternative. Desensitization is a process that allows transplantation in highly sensitized and ABO incompatible donor and recipient. Researchers initially developed principles of desensitization for kidney transplantation and have subsequently applied them to other types of solid organ transplantation. Desensitization protocols vary by the transplant center, but most use combinations of apheresis, intravenous immunoglobulin (IVIG), and anti-CD20 monoclonal antibodies. The desensitization aims to ease the immunological détente by removing preformed donor-specific alloantibodies (DSA) and creating a favorable immune environment for the allograft. Desensitization caries risk; therefore, careful patient selection and close monitoring are essential to mitigate the risk of complications. Further work is required to enhance the outcomes of desensitization.

Keywords: desensitization, calculated PRA, HLA incompatible, ABO incompatible, solid organ transplantation

1. Introduction

Solid organ transplantation is the optimal treatment for selected patients with end-stage organ disorders. Two important immunologic barriers to SOT are HLA sensitization and ABO incompatibility. The options for transplant candidates with incompatible donors are prioritization to well-matched organs in the allocation system, such as acceptable mismatch and paired donation programs or desensitization. Experience from renal transplantation forms the basis of contemporary desensitization protocols in SOT. This chapter will discuss desensitization in HLA incompatible (HLAi) and ABO incompatible renal transplantation. A brief account of desensitization in cardiac and lung transplantation is also provided.

2. HLAi renal transplantation

Antibodies against HLA are critical immunologic barriers to successful transplantation. The formation of HLA antibodies before or after transplantation is associated with poor graft and patient outcomes [1].

In the United States, 35% of waitlisted renal transplant candidates are sensitized. Fifteen percent of them are highly sensitized with calculated panel reactive antibodies (cPRA) >80% [2]. HLA sensitization restricts the number of compatible donors, thus reducing the chances of finding an acceptable HLA phenotype donor. Currently, only 6.5% of highly sensitized patients (cPRA > 80%) receive renal transplants each year [3]. Data from the United Network of Organ Sharing (UNOS) show longer waiting time for transplantation in sensitized individuals [4] (**Table 1**). Furthermore, sensitization increases the risk of hyper-acute, accelerated, and chronic graft rejection post-transplantation.

Highly sensitized individuals have three options to access renal transplantation, i.e., either,

- Wait till a negative crossmatch donor becomes available, but this may take years OR,
- Consider paired kidney donation, but the chances of finding an appropriate donor are comparatively low OR,
- Undergo HLA incompatible transplantation with desensitization.

Desensitization reduces the cPRA by reducing DSA levels and thus increases the chances of getting an organ from a compatible donor. Furthermore, it lowers the risk of hyperacute rejection post-transplantation.

3. Essential concepts and terminology of transplant immunology

3.1 What are human leucocyte antigens (HLA)?

HLA are glycoproteins expressed on the cell surface that differentiate between 'self' and 'non-self' antigens. The primary purpose of HLA is to combat pathogens [5], but it poses a crucial barrier to transplantation.

The human major histocompatibility complex (MHC) on the short arm of chromosome 6 encodes HLA. They are the most polymorphic genes in the human genome. There are currently 37,068 HLA and related alleles in the human genome, and it is

cPRA level (%)	Renal transplant candidates waiting for >5 yrs (%)
<80	8.8
80–89	10.7
90–98	17
99	20.9

Table 1.
Association of cPRA level and waiting time to renal transplantation.

growing [6]. Antigen presenting cells present foreign antigens *via* MHC proteins to the T cells, which switch on the host immune system.

MHC encodes two classes of antigens, i.e., class I, which includes HLA-A, B, and C antigenic clusters and class II antigens comprising HLA-DQ, DP, and DR clusters [7]. Class I antigens are expressed on nucleated cells, platelets, and red blood cells (in ~15% of individuals). Class II antigens are expressed on antigen-presenting cells, e.g., macrophages, B cells, and dendritic cells. However, other cells, e.g., epithelial and endothelial cells, can express class II antigens during inflammatory states, e.g., infections [8].

3.2 HLA typing

HLA typing is performed to assess HLA mismatches between the donor and recipient. Preformed DSA are also measured at this stage. HLA mismatch exists when an HLA antigen is present in the donor but not in the recipient. The higher the mismatches, the more foreign the graft is immunologically and is likely to mount an immune response.

Historically, typing has focused on HLA-A, HLA-B, HLA-DQ, and HLA-DR loci in renal transplantation. The reason for emphasizing on these loci was that the DSAs against these antigens pose a significant risk of hyperacute and accelerated rejection; however, typing limitations also had a role.

Serological assays were used to type HLA initially. However, it is now replaced by DNA-based molecular techniques, which include sequence-specific priming (SSP), real-time PCR, and reverse sequence-specific oligonucleotide probing (rSSOP).

3.3 What is HLA sensitization?

The presence of HLA-specific antibodies in an individual's serum defines HLA sensitization. HLA antibodies directed against the donor HLA are called donor specific antibodies (DSA). Sensitization occurs through blood transfusion, pregnancy, and transplantation. **Table 2** illustrates the variation in the vigor of the alloimmune response to the type of sensitizing event [9, 10]. Proinflammatory conditions like infections and trauma influence the strength and breadth of the HLA antibodies [11].

Positive complement-dependent crossmatch (CDCXM) or flow cytometer crossmatch (FCXM) before transplantation defines HLAi transplantation. Class I DSA is associated with acute rejection, while class II DSA causes chronic rejection [12, 13].

3.4 DSA screening and cross match

DSA screening is performed using cell-based crossmatch and solid phase techniques. Due to the limitations of the cell-based assays, most HLA laboratories have moved to more advanced assays.

Sensitization event	HLA seroconversion rate	Median fluorescence index (MFI)
Previous transplantation	50–75%	14,164
Pregnancy	38.3%	4185
Blood transfusion	20–33%	5548

Table 2.
HLA seroconversion rates after various sensitization events.

Solid phase multiplex assays have significantly improved the detection of anti-HLA DSA. It is performed by incubating the recipient's serum with the polystyrene beads to which purified HLA antigens are attached. Then, a florescent conjugated IgG antibody is added. Flow cytometer or Luminex reads the test results.

Most laboratories will first perform screening using beads with multiple HLA antigens. If the screening test is positive, then a single antigen bead (SAB) assay is performed to detect the specificity of the antibody. SAB assay is a semiquantitative measure and can identify only anti-HLA IgG DSA. The output of the assay is expressed as mean or median fluorescence intensity (MFI). It represents the strength and amount of the DSA. A standardized cut-off MFI value above which the result is reported positive is not clearly defined. Each laboratory sets its cut-off point. A study reported >90% consensus among the HLA laboratories for MFI positive cut-off range of 1000–1500 [14]. MFI > 5000 is considered cytotoxic by most.

Despite the improved sensitivity of solid-phase technology, it has certain limitations and cell-based assays are still in use. False positive results can occur due to denatured proteins on the beads. C1q and complement products could bind to the beads, thus obscuring antibody detection (prozone effect) [15]. Similarly, IgM antibodies or intravenous immunoglobulins could hinder IgG binding to the beads, thus giving a false negative result. This effect could be countered by using ethylene diamine tetraacetic acid (EDTA), dithiothreitol (DDT), or heat inactivation [16, 17]. Antibodies against public epitopes bind with more than one bead, causing an underestimation of the true DSA. Renal transplant candidates with no history of sensitization and little or no DSA detection on solid phase assay do not require further investigations.

Due to technical reasons, many laboratories are transitioning away from cell-based crossmatches. However, despite this shift, it is still performed in specific situations. Two types of cell-based cross matches are available.

Complement-dependent cytotoxicity crossmatch (CDCXM) assay is performed by mixing the recipient's serum with donor lymphocytes (T and B). Then, an exogenous complement and a viability dye are added. Suppose a complement binding DSA is present in the recipient's serum. In that case, it will bind to the HLA antigens on the donor lymphocyte, which activates complement and causes cell lysis, rendering the test positive. A positive T cell CDCXM identifies class I antibodies, and a positive B cell crossmatch indicates antibodies against class I and II antigens.

Flow cytometry crossmatch (FCXM) assay is more sensitive and detects IgG DSA regardless of its ability to activate complement [18]. Like CDCXM, FCXM is performed by mixing the donor's lymphocytes with the recipient's sera. The flow cytometer reads the analysis results and expresses them as the median fluorescence index (MFI). The presence of DSA is determined by channel shift of fluorescence intensity beyond a pre-determined value.

Cell-based crossmatch techniques require live donor cells and have low precision in detecting the specificity of anti-HLA antibodies. Non-HLA antibodies (including autoimmune antibodies) can give false positive results. Therefore, an autologous crossmatch is performed when a cell-based crossmatch assay is positive to evaluate the presence of autoantibodies. Low titer DSA may be unable to activate the complement pathway and missed. This deficiency could be improved by using anti-human globulin (AHG) which, amplifies complement activation. AHG also helps in differentiating complement and non-complement binding DSAs. IgM HLA and non-HLA antibodies can cause false positive crossmatch. Cell-based assays are not standardized, and therefore, inter-laboratory variations exist. Furthermore, these assays are time-consuming prolonging cold ischemia time and affect organ sharing [19].

A tool called panel reactive antibodies (PRA) measures the degree of sensitization. Previously, PRA was determined using cell-based assays; however, United Network for Organ Sharing (UNOS) mandated to replace it with calculated PRA (cPRA) in 2007. cPRA is based on SAB assays. This tool provides HLA antibody specificity in combination with HLA antigen frequencies in the donor population. For example, a patient with DSA against HLA B44 (which is reported in 27% of the United States donors), will have 27% cPRA. Put differently, this patient will not be able to get organ from 27% of the donors.

The degree of sensitization is not precisely defined; however, most centers consider cPRA of 0–10% non-sensitized and >80% highly sensitized.

Virtual crossmatch (VCXM) provides valuable information about the risk of antibody-mediated rejection (ABMR) using the recipient's DSA against the donor HLA typing without running an actual crossmatch. Virtual crossmatch (VCXM) is considered positive when a DSA occurs at a cut-off value above the acceptable or manageable level [19]. Virtual crossmatch accurately predicts the outcomes of FCXM in >85% of the cases [20], but the correlation with CDCXM is low due to the higher sensitivity of solid phase assays. The negative predictive value of VCXM is high for early ABMR. In sensitized patients, the error rate of VCXM is 15%; therefore, actual crossmatch is still required for risk stratification. VCXM has shortened timelines for organ allocation in heart, lung, and kidney transplantation [19, 21]. Actual crossmatch could be omitted in non-sensitized recipients with no history of sensitization and negative VCXM. An incomplete donor HLA profile diminishes the accuracy of virtual crossmatch.

3.5 Integration of immune data for risk assessment

Integrating data from multiple immunologic tests provides a better idea of the risk, as illustrated in **Table 3**.

4. Outcomes of desensitization in HLAi renal transplantation

4.1 Patient and graft survival

The outcome data of HLAi renal transplantation is contradictory. Two retrospective studies from the United States compared patient survival after HLAi renal transplant to waitlist and transplanted population. **Table 4** illustrates the results.

In contrast to the above data, a retrospective study of HLAi renal transplantation from the UK did not show a significant difference in patient survival compared to those who continued dialysis while waiting for transplant or got transplanted ($p = 0.98$) and waitlisted only ($p = 0.44$) [22]. Controls were matched for age, sex, cPRA, blood group, diabetes mellitus as the primary cause of ESRD, number of previous transplants, duration on paired kidney donation list, and ESRD vintage. Positive CDCXM or FCXM defined HLA incompatibility. The author excluded patients with negative crossmatch but positive DSA.

Another study, including 326 highly sensitized patients (>80% PRA), examined patient survival [23]. Thirty-six patients were desensitized with rituximab and plasmapheresis. Thirty patients received kidney transplants. One hundred forty-nine patients were transplanted without desensitization, and 141 remained on dialysis. The investigators did not observe significant differences in mortality among the groups ($HR = 0.48$, $p = 0.22$).

CDCXM		FCXM		HLA antibody type	Interpretation
B cell	T cell	B cell	T cell		
Current tests					
+	+	+	+	IgG class I DSA	• High risk for HAR • Tx absolute contraindicated
+	—	+	—	IgG class II DSA	• High risk for accelerated/refractory ABMR and poor long-term outcomes • Tx contraindicated in most centers
+	—	+	—	IgG weak class I DSA	• High risk for accelerated/refractory ABMR and poor long-term outcomes • Tx contraindicated in most centers
—	—	+	+	IgG class I DSA	• High risk for accelerated/refractory ABMR and poor long-term outcomes • Tx contraindicated in most centers
—	—	+	—	IgG class II DSA	Intermediate risk. Consider PKD or desensitization
Historical tests					
+	+	+	+	IgG class I DSA	High risk
+	—	+	—	IgG class II DSA	High risk
+	—	+	—	IgG weak class I DSA	Intermediate risk. Consider PKD or desensitization
—	—	+	+	IgG class I DSA	Intermediate risk. Consider PKD or desensitization
—	—	+	—	IgG class II DSA	Intermediate risk. Consider PKD or desensitization
Current or historical					
—	—	—	—	IgG class I or II DSA	Low risk
—	—	+	+	HLA antibody but no DSA	Low risk
+	+	+	+	Negative	Low risk. Autoreactive non-HLA IgG/IgM

Table 3.
Immunological risk assessment in renal transplant candidate.

Author	Study group	1 yr (%)	3 yr (%)	4 yr (%)	8 yr (%)
Montgomery et al. [15]	HLAi renal Tx	90.6	85.7	80.6	80.6
	Wait listed dialysis or transplantation	93.1	77	65.6	49.1
	Wait listed only	91.1	67.2	51.5	30.5
Orandi et al. [22]	HLAi renal Tx	95	91.7	86	76.5
	Wait listed dialysis or transplantation	94	83.6	74.4	62.9
	Wait listed only	89	72.7	59.2	43.9

Table 4.
Patient survival post renal transplant with desensitization.

Another study, including 372 desensitized recipients, showed no difference in patient or graft survival over 60 months among the study groups [24].

The reasons for contradictory results between the United States and Europe are unknown. However, the survival rate on dialysis therapy in the United States is comparatively lower.

Table 5 summarizes graft and patient outcome data from other studies.

4.2 Acute rejection

The risk of acute rejection is higher in HLAi renal transplants than in HLA-compatible, living donor transplants (21 vs. 8%) [36]. The risk increases proportionality with the degree of incompatibility. Acute rejection occurred in 18% of patients with DSA but negative FCXM, 21% with positive FCXM but negative CDCXM, and 22% with positive CDCXM. Interestingly, most of the rejections were ABMR [24].

4.3 Infectious complications

The data about the risk of infection after desensitization is contradictory. A retrospective study compared infections in HLAi and ABOi to compatible transplant recipients. There was no significant difference in the infection rates between the groups after 18 months [25]. On the contrary, a Korean organ Transplant registry study reported a higher rate of infections in the HLAi and ABOi transplantation (89 vs. 27%) [26].

A European study reported a higher rate of deaths from infection in the first year after ABOi transplants [27].

Author	Desensitization protocol	n=	ABMR (%)	F/U period (yr)	Graft survival (%)	Patient survival (%)
Tyan et al. [25]	High dose IVIG	15	6	1	81.8	100
Montgomery et al. [26]	PP + low dose IVIG + Rituximab	211	NR	1	>90	90.6
Guthoff et al. [27]	PP + low dose IVIG + Eculizumab	16	NR	1	100	100
Thielki et al. [28]	PP + low dose IVIG	51	24	2	81	91
Jordan et al. [29]	High dose IVIG + Rituximab	76	NR	2	84	95
Al Meshari et al. [30]	PP + IVIG	124	4	2	96	98
Klein et al. [31]	PP or IA + Rituximab	23	22	2	100	100
Jin et al. [32]	PP + low dose IVIG + Rituximab	6	0	2.7	100	100
Kahwaji et al. [33]	High dose IVIG	79	8	3	87.1	97.5
Warren et al. [34]	PP + low dose IVIG + splenectomy/PP + high dose IVIG/high dose IVIG alone/no Tx	102	31	5	70.7	83.5
Bentall et al. [35]	PP + low dose IVIG/PP + high dose IVIG/high dose IVIG alone	102	37.2	5	70.7	92.5

Table 5.
Graft and patient survival after HLAi transplantation.

Data about malignancy risk in HLAi renal transplants is limited. The risk of malignancy in ABOi renal transplants is like that of ABO-compatible transplants.

4.4 Cost of HLAi Tx

An HLAi renal transplant costs more than an HLA-compatible transplant due to pre-transplant conditioning, longer hospitalization, monitoring, and frequent biopsies. The mean cost of a HLAi renal transplant was $151,024 compared to $106,306 in a matched control study [28]. The price increases incrementally with the degree of incompatibility.

Prospective studies are required to analyze the quality of life and morbidity associated with desensitization.

5. Desensitization regimens

Desensitization aims to increase access to kidney transplantation in broadly sensitized individuals and to prevent ABMR after transplantation. In renal transplantation, desensitization could be done in a living or deceased donor setup. However, it is only performed in the deceased donor settings in heart and lung transplantation due to the nature of the donor and the organ transplanted.

In the living donor scenario, desensitization is planned well before surgery. In the deceased donor program, desensitization is attempted in the pre and peri-transplant period.

The desensitization protocols vary from center to center. Consensus is lacking on a standardized desensitization protocol among renal the transplant community. Most protocols use the following interventions in combinations (**Table 6**).

5.1 Immunoglobulin (IVIG)

IVIG predominantly contains IgG (90-99%) from pooled human plasma. The exact mechanism of action of IVIG is unknown; however, it exerts immunomodulatory effects via multiple pathways. It blocks the FC receptors on plasma cells, thus preventing the rebound of DSA. Furthermore, blocking the FC neonatal receptor increases the lysosomal degradation of the circulating IgG [29]. Some researchers previously reported hemolysis with high-dose IVIG administration [30]. It was linked with the presence of anti-A/B isohemagglutinins [31]. It led to improvements in IVIG manufacturing, and the modern formulations carry a low risk of hemolysis [32].

High-dose IVIG (2 g/kg) alone enabled renal transplantation in 13/15 highly sensitized patients in a study [33]. In another study, 2 g/kg IVIG was administered before and after renal and heart transplantation in 45 CDCXM positive candidates [34].

Mechanism	Intervention
Immunomodulation	Immunoglobulins (IVIG)
Antibody depletion	Plasmapheresis or adsorption
B cell depletion	Rituximab

Table 6.
Therapeutic agents for desensitization in renal transplantation.

Crossmatch became negative in 35 cases and reduced to positive FCXM in the remaining seven candidates. Forty-two candidates were transplanted eventually. Acute rejection occurred in 31% of cases, and 7% lost graft. At 24 months, 89% had a functioning graft. Investigators from Cedar Sinai Center reported successful renal transplantation in highly sensitized candidates using high-dose IVIG and induction therapy [35, 37, 38]. Graft outcomes varied according to immunologic risk. Graft survival was 94–96% and 40–100% at 1 and 2 years, respectively. Fifteen to 35% of cases experienced ABMR.

A randomized trial of 48 sensitized individuals (PRA > 50%) compared high-dose IVIG for 4 months to placebo [39]. IVIG shortened the time to transplantation from 10.3 to 4.8 years. Thirty-five percent of candidates in the intervention group received transplants compared to 17% in the control group. Rejections occurred in 53% of cases in the IVIG group while 10% in the control group. Graft survival was 80% in the IVIG group and 75% in the control group at 30 months.

5.2 Apheresis

Apheresis has been part of desensitization regimens since the 1990s [40]. Apheresis removes preformed antibodies from the plasma. Various apheresis modalities are used in desensitization though the ideal apheresis technique in desensitization is not known yet. **Table 7** compares various apheresis modalities. A single-center, retrospective study looked at different apheresis modalities [41] in 45 DSA-positive renal transplant candidates. All modalities decreased DSA, but immunoadsorption (IA) and plasma exchange (PE) were more efficient than double filtration plasmapheresis (DFPP). DFPP is associated with severe adverse events, e.g., hypotension, high leukocyte counts, and low fibrinogen levels.

IA is frequently used in Europe, while PE is standard in the United States. Bleeding complications are more frequent with PE [42]. Giving time for fibrinogen to return to normal or repletion with cryoprecipitate before surgery reduces the risk of bleeding.

A retrospective case-control study compared desensitization with PE (1–12 sessions) + IVIG (100 mg/kg) in FCXM-positive renal transplant recipients to FCXM-negative controls [43]. Graft loss was high in the FCXM positive group at 9-year (14 vs. 7) [HR 2.6 (95% CI 1.03–6.4) $t^{1/2}$ = 6.8 yr.] Graft survival at 1 and 5 years were 89.9 and 69.4% in the FCXM positive group compared to 97.6 and 80.6% in the control group. In conclusion, the medium- and long-term outcomes of positive FCXM living

	Plasma exchange (PE)	Double filtration plasmapheresis (DFPP)	Immunoadsorption (IA)
Duration	2 hrs	3–4 hrs	6–8 hrs
Plasma volume processed	1–1.5	1–2	2–3
Substitution solution	+++	+	—
Removal of coagulation factors	++++	++	—
Selectivity for antibody removal	+	++	++++

Table 7.
Comparison of plasmapheresis techniques.

Pre-transplant desensitization regimen (n=)	Achieving negative cross match (%)	ABMR at 6 weeks (%)
High dose IVIG alone (n = 13)	36	80
PE + low dose IVIG + rituximab (n = 32)	84	37
PE + low dose IVIG + rituximab + pre-transplant ATG + DSA monitoring (n = 16)	88	29

Table 8.
Summary of study outcomes.

kidney recipients are not promising. The results are comparable to extended criteria deceased donor renal transplantation.

A prospective study compared IVIG alone with two different combinations of PE, IVIG, and other interventions (**Table 8**) [44]. The author concluded that PE regimens result in lower ABMRs than IVIG-only regimens. Moreover, despite achieving a negative crossmatch, the rejection rate remained high in all the groups.

A pilot study analyzed the efficacy of two desensitization regimens in sensitized kidney transplant candidates who received deceased donor grafts [45]. The results (shown in **Table 9**) illustrate that intense immunosuppression on day 0 could improve long-term graft outcomes.

Another retrospective case-control study (n = 48) examined five desensitization protocols [46]. The participants were stratified into five based on the MFI levels of the immunodominant DSA. Acute ABMR (25 vs. 12.5%) and T cell mediate rejection (TCMR) (23 vs. 14%) were high in desensitized recipients. However, graft loss and patient survival were similar across the groups.

5.3 Anti-CD-20 therapies

Rituximab is a chimeric anti-CD20 monoclonal antibody. FDA initially approved it for lymphoma; however, it plays a role in autoimmune disorders and SOT. A combination of rituximab (1 gm on day 7 and 22) and high-dose IVIG (on day 0 and 30) showed a significant reduction in PRA (44 vs. 77%) in Phase I/II trial (n = 20) [38]. Although the ABMR rate was high at 31%, graft survival was 94% at 1 year.

In another study, the investigators desensitized 76 highly sensitized patients with rituximab and IVIG combination [37]. PRA declined significantly from 79.7 ± 25.6% to 67.1 ± 28.6% for class I and 59.7 ± 29.2% to 49.7 ± 27.8% for class II anti-HLA

Desensitization regimen	Acute ABMR (%)	Microcirculation inflammation at 1 yr	Transplant glomerulopathy rate at 1 yr (%)	Chronic ABMR rate at 1 yr	eGFR at 1 year (ml/min/1.73 m^2)
IVIG (2 g/kg on day 0, 21, 42 and 63) [n = 36]	19.6	2.7 ± 0.2	38	41.1	43 ± 16
IVIG (2 g/kg) + PE (9.8 ± 4) + rituximab (375 mg/m^2 on day 4) [n = 18]	16.6	1.8 ± 0.2	7	13.3	54 ± 16

Table 9.
Study result summary.

antibodies. Fifty-nine percent of the participants received deceased donor kidney transplants. Graft survival was 84% at 24 months, but the ABMR rate was high at 37%.

A combination of rituximab and high-dose IVIG enabled renal transplantation in 71% of candidates in another study [47]. Transplantation with desensitization was more cost-effective than continuing dialysis.

A retrospective study compared desensitization with plasmapheresis and low-dose IVIG combination with or without rituximab (375 mg/m^2) [48]. The rebound of DSA and non-DSA anti-HLA antibodies were lower with the rituximab group (7 and 33% respectively) compared to the no rituximab group (32 and 55% respectively) at 1-month post-transplantation. However, rituximab did not alter the ABMR rate, 5-year allograft survival, and elimination of HLA antibodies.

A randomized control trial compared high-dose IVIG + rituximab (1 g) with high-dose IVIG + placebo in sensitized renal transplant candidates [49]. Six patients in the intervention and seven in the placebo arm received deceased donor kidney transplants. DSA levels at transplantation were not different, but ABMR was seen only in the placebo arm. No graft loss occurred in the rituximab arm compared to 2 in the placebo arm. The study was prematurely stopped due to poor outcomes in the placebo arm.

Obinutuzumab is a type II anti-CD20 monoclonal antibody used in refractory and relapsing hematological malignancies. It is more efficient than rituximab in depleting B-cells in lymphoid organs. An open-label phase I trial (n = 25) assessed the efficacy of obinutuzumab + IVIG (2 g/kg) in sensitized renal transplant candidates [50]. MFI levels decreased significantly but were clinically irrelevant. Nine patients developed severe adverse events, mainly infectious complications. Though encouraging, these results need further validation.

In summary, the combination of apheresis + IVIG and or B cell-depleting agent is the most used desensitization protocol in renal transplantation.

The exact sequence and doses of the desensitization therapies vary among the centers. We perform low and intermediate risk living donor HLAi incompatible renal transplants at our center. We do not perform CDCXM positive transplants. Low risk HLAi renal transplant candidates (DSA positive but negative FCXM) are desensitized with 1 gram/ kg single IVIG dose. Patients with intermediate risk HLAi renal transplants [DSA positive and FCXM positive (≤300 median channel shift)] receive a single dose of rituximab 500 mg IV with pre-medications a week before transplantation. Two doses of IVIG 1 gram/kg/day (max dose 140 gm) are administered on subsequent days. PE or IA is not used in HLAi transplant desensitization at our center. We do not repeat FCXM after desensitization therapy.

In deceased donor kidney transplantation, due to the unpredictable timing of the organ availability, pre-transplant desensitization is offered only to those within 1 year of receiving renal grafts. High-dose IVIG and rituximab are given in the same protocol as the living donors. Luminex single antigen testing is performed monthly to maintain the current sera for crossmatch testing. A second course of desensitization, consisting of PE sessions followed by high-dose IVIG and rituximab, is offered if a patient does not receive a transplant within six months. PE (1.5 plasma volume with 5% albumin replacement) is performed on alternate days. IVIG 2 gram/kg (maximum dose of 140 g) is delivered immediately following the last plasmapheresis session. Rituximab 375 mg/m^2 is given one week after the last PE and IVIG session to avoid IVIG saturation of the Fc receptors [51]. This protocol is repeated every 6 months until the patient receives a transplant.

5.4 Alternative approaches

Bortezomib is a reversible proteasome inhibitor. It induces apoptosis of the differentiated plasma cells. A retrospective study of 44 sensitized patients (PRA > 20%) with positive CDCXM or a FCXM were desensitized with 1–2 cycles of bortezomib 1.3 mg/m^2 (6–8 doses) + rituximab (375 mg/m^2) and plasmapheresis [52]. Nineteen patients received kidney grafts from living donors. Immunodominant DSA declined 51.1% in 83% of the cases. ABMR rate was 12.5%, and graft survival was 94.7% at 1.2 yr.

In another study, 32 doses of bortezomib 1.3 mg/m^2 alone were administered for desensitization in 10 highly sensitized renal transplant candidates. Although MFI values declined after bortezomib, crossmatch, and cPRA remained unchanged [53]. Two patients discontinued therapy due to side effects and two had to reduce the dose.

Carfilzomib is an irreversible proteasome inhibitor. It has a sustained and durable effect on plasma cells compared to bortezomib. Furthermore, it has better tolerability than bortezomib. A combination of 12 escalating doses of carflizomib (20–32 mg/m^2) + PE (minimum three sessions) was trialed in 13 sensitized patients (mean PRA 97%) [54]. The immunodominant DSA declined by >50% in 70% of cases; however, the antibodies rebounded within 5 months after treatment discontinuation.

Eculizumab is a humanized monoclonal antibody against terminal complement component C5. It is used in ABMR treatment; however, experience in desensitization is limited. Thirty renal transplant candidates with initial B cell positive crossmatch (mean channel shift 200–450) were administered 1200 mg eculizumab immediately before transplantation, followed by 600 mg weekly dose for 4 weeks [55]. Patients with mean channel shift >300 were treated with plasmapheresis before transplantation to bring it down to <300. The outcomes were compared with a historical control who received the same desensitization protocol but without eculizumab. ABMR incidence was low in the eculizumab group, but the DSA rebounded.

A study compared the C1-inhibitor to placebo as a desensitization agent. Twenty highly sensitized patients (PRA > 50% and positive FCXM) who received plasmapheresis + rituximab + IVIG were randomized to C1-inhibitor or placebo [56]. ABMR was low in the intervention arm (20 vs. 30%, $p = 0.6$). Further validation is needed.

5.5 Investigational agents

Imlifidase is a recombinant IgG endopeptidase produced by *Streptococcus pyogenes*. It cleaves all sub-classes of IgG into Fc and F (ab) fragments. European Medicine Agency (EMA) has granted conditional approval for Imlifidase in desensitization, but the US Food and Drug Administration (FDA) is yet to approve it.

Two independent phase I/II studies (n = 25) were conducted in the United States and Sweden in highly sensitized patients (cPRA 96% and 81% respectively) [57]. Eight percent of participants had positive FCXM, and 92% had DSA. Imlifidase (0.24 mg/kg in the USA and 0.25 mg/kg or 0.5 mg/kg in Sweden) was given to all patients 4-6 hours pre-transplant. Ninety-two percent of the candidates received deceased donor kidney transplants. The United States cohort received a high dose IVIG, rituximab, and alemtuzumab at induction, while the Swedish population received horse ATG at induction but no IVIG and rituximab. IgG antibodies in the recipient serums were cleaved within 6 hours of the infusion and remained absent for at least 7 days. IgG recovered gradually but remained low at 28 days after the infusion.

DSA rebounded in the Swedish cohort between 7 and 14 days. In the United States cohort, DSA rebound was low. One patient from the US cohort had hyperacute rejection attributable to IgM DSA. The ABMR rate was 27% in the Swedish cohort at two weeks, while only 14% experienced ABMR at 2 and 5 months in the US cohort. Mean GFR at 1–6 months was 70 and 49 ml/min/1.73 m^2 in the United States and Swedish cohorts, respectively.

Another multinational phase II study assessed the crossmatch conversion efficacy of Imlifidase in 19 highly sensitized kidney transplant candidates [58]. Eighty-nine percent (n = 17/19) of patients achieved a negative crossmatch within 24 hours of treatment. Thirteen patients received deceased donor kidney transplants, five received a living donor transplant, and one patient was not considered for transplantation due to a reaction to Imlifidase. DSA rebounded within 3–14 days after the treatment, though MFIs were lower than the pre-transplant level. Patient and graft survival at six months was 100% and 89%, respectively. Half of the patients experienced acute rejection; most (7/9) were ABMR.

A retrospective study examined 3 years of follow-up data of 39 crossmatch positive patients who received renal transplants [59]. Thirty-eight percent (n = 15/39) experienced ABMR. Overall graft survival was 84% at 3 years, notably lower in those who experienced ABMR (77 vs. 93%). Imlifidase has shown promising results, but further research is needed.

Clazakizumab- is a humanized, anti-interleukin (IL)-6 monoclonal antibody. It is used in chronic active ABMR in kidney transplantation, but experience as a desensitization agent is limited. Twenty highly sensitized patients (mean cPRA 96%) were desensitized with plasmapheresis, high-dose IVIG, and clazakizumab (25 mg * 6 doses) in a pilot study [60]. Eighteen patients received deceased donor renal transplants. Clazakizumab was continued for 12 months post-transplantation. MFI levels declined in almost all patients. Rejection occurred in four cases; one graft was lost due to a technical problem. Patient survival was 100 percent at the end of the study. Further studies are needed to validate these findings.

Belimumab is a human monoclonal antibody that inhibits B cell activating factor. However, it failed to show notable results in a pilot study as a desensitization agent [61]. Similarly, Atacicept, another monoclonal antibody targeting B cell activating factor, did not achieve the desired results in pre-clinical desensitization studies [62, 63].

Daratumumab (anti-CD38 antibody) and anti-C-X-C chemokine receptor type 4 decreased DSA in animal models and improved graft survival [64]. Validation in clinical trials is awaited.

5.6 Post renal transplant monitoring

Monitoring protocols vary from center to center. Some centers monitor HLAi renal transplant recipients like HLA compatible patients but keep a low threshold for renal biopsy in case of graft dysfunction. Other centers prefer protocol renal biopsies at pre-defined time points. Most centers monitor DSA after HLAi transplantation, though the frequency of monitoring varies. In our center, DSA are monitored monthly for the first 3 months, every 3 months up to 12 months, and then yearly. IVIG given during the pre-conditioning therapy could show false positive DSA due to non-specific binding of IVIG to SAB, but this effect fades away after 2 months. Renal biopsy is performed in patients with persistent de novo DSA to rule out ABMR.

6. Blood type incompletable (ABOi) renal transplantation

Blood type or ABO incompatibility (ABOi) poses another barrier to SOT. Earlier attempts to cross the ABO barrier without desensitization failed [65]. It was an absolute contraindication for transplantation due to the higher risk of ABMR and graft failure. However, the shortage of deceased organ availability (especially in Japan) fueled the re-exploration of this avenue. Moreover, approximately one-third of the living donors have ABOi with their potential recipients. ABOi renal transplants are performed globally thanks to desensitization. The outcomes of ABOi renal transplants are comparable to ABO-compatible transplants [66].

Blood group antigens are present on red blood cells, platelets, lymphocytes, endothelial cells, and epithelial cells. Human blood is classified into four blood groups, i.e., A, B, AB and O. Blood group antibodies called isohemagglutinins, are formed against non-self-blood group antigens. For example, an individual with blood group A will have antibodies against B antigens, while a person with blood group O will have antibodies to both A and B antigens.

Blood group O donors can donate to any blood group. In contrast, blood group AB recipients can receive grafts from all blood group types without desensitization. The blood type frequencies in the population vary; however, blood groups A and O are the most common. Renal transplant candidates with blood groups O and B wait longer on the waiting list for compatible donors. In the context of ABOi transplantation, both IgM and IgG isohemagglutinins are clinically relevant.

It is also important to note that individuals with the blood group O produce higher Isohemagglutinins levels than those with blood type A or B. Therefore, the risk of ABMR is higher with blood type O after ABOi transplantation.

Blood type A consists of two sub-groups: A1 and non-A1. A1 type occurs in 80% of the population, while non-A1 is observed in 20% of the US population. The non-A1 type carries low immunologic risk due to lower antigenic expression.

The measurement and reporting of ABO isohemagglutinin vary from center to center [67]. Isohemagglutinins titers are measured by the dilution method. Interpretation of this method is observer-dependent, and the outcomes are semi-quantitative. For example, the actual value of isohemagglutinins titer 1:8 could range between 1:4 and 1:32. Some centers use column agglutination technology, but it is expensive.

6.1 Desensitization in ABOi renal transplantation

The purpose of ABO desensitization is to reduce pre-transplant anti-A/B isohemagglutinins, reducing the risk of ABMR, and allowing successful transplantation. ABO desensitization therapy is commenced well before the transplant surgery. It is offered presently in the living donor set up only. However, sporadic cases of deceased donor ABOi renal transplants are reported [68, 69]. There is a lack of consensus about a standard ABOi desensitization protocol. Therefore, protocols are center specific. However, like HLAi transplantation, most centers use the following treatments in various combinations,

- Aphaeresis—The risk of acute ABMR is high in patients with higher pre-transplant isoagglutinin titers [70]. Apheresis reduces the circulating anti-A/B isohemagglutinins to a predetermined titer. Most protocols consider isohemagglutinins titers (IgG and IgM) ≤ 1:8 safe for transplantation. Some centers perform transplantation with isohemagglutinins titers up to 1:32 [71]. Most centers decline candidates for transplantation with baseline isohemagglutinins titers ≥1:256 for both IgM and IgG using the tube dilution method. One PE session (1.5 plasma volume) reduces isohemagglutinins titer by one dilution. The baseline isohemagglutinins titers help in calculating the dose and frequency of apheresis.

- IVIG- Most centers administer low-dose IVIG (100 mg/kg) after each apheresis to replace the eliminated immunoglobulins. Moreover, it also causes immunomodulation, as explained in section 4.1.

- Splenectomy and B cell depleting agent—Before the rituximab era, splenectomy was part of the ABOi desensitization protocol [72]. Nowadays, splenectomy is rarely practiced, thanks to the introduction of rituximab.

ABO desensitization therapy is commenced before the scheduled surgery date; however, the time and sequence of desensitization therapy varies according to the center.

In our center, a single rituximab dose (500 mg IV) is administered with premedications 2 weeks before surgery. PE is initiated 1 week before the operation. Each exchange is followed by a 100 mg/kg IVIG replacement. Three doses of ATG (1.5 mg/kg/day) are administered at induction. Patients are maintained on a triple maintenance regimen. A/B isohemagglutinins titers are checked daily for 2 weeks. After a fortnight, the allograft develops immunologic accommodation to low levels of A/B isohemagglutinins and resists complement-mediated damage. Additional PE and renal biopsy are considered with rising isohemagglutinins titers and serum creatinine levels within the first two weeks. Some units commence desensitization and maintenance immunosuppression simultaneously a month before the scheduled surgery. PE has not been considered in some centers if A/B isohemagglutinins titers are ≤1:16 [73], but higher rejection rates are reported with this practice.

There is a lack of high-quality evidence to guide optimal desensitization protocol for ABOi renal transplantation; however, non-randomized studies data show the efficacy of the combination therapies described above. Plasma exchange and immunoadsorption effectively remove isohemagglutinins [74]. Although IVIG is used in most ABOi desensitization protocols, this practice has not been trialed in randomized studies. Moreover, the optimal dose of IVIG is also not clearly defined. Rituximab and splenectomy are not directly studied. A systematic review showed similar graft and patient survival comparing splenectomy-based and rituximab-based protocols [75]. Some researchers have reported successful ABOi renal transplantation without using rituximab; however, they employed daily plasmapheresis for at least 2 weeks to keep isohemagglutinins titers ≤1:16 [76].

6.2 Outcomes and cost of ABOi renal transplantation

The risk of complications is high in the first few years after ABOi renal transplantation. A meta-analysis reported higher mortality in the first 3 years after an ABOi transplant vs. ABO compatible renal transplant [77]. However, this difference fails to exist at 8 years or more. Similarly, death-censored graft survival was low in ABOi vs. ABO compatible transplants, but this difference equalizes after 5 years. Furthermore, the risk of surgical complications, rejection, infections, and malignancy is higher in ABOi compared to ABO-compatible transplants.

The outcomes of ABOi and HLAi transplants are inferior to compatible transplants. However, desensitization is justified in selected patients due to long waiting time, high mortality on dialysis and low access to compatible donors.

ABOi renal transplantation bears a higher monetary cost. The average total cost of hospitalization was $65,080 for ABOi vs. $32,039 for compatible transplants [78]. However, the benefits of ABOi transplants outweigh its higher cost in the long run. Due to suboptimal outcomes, efforts should be made to avoid ABO incompatible transplantation; however, if it is not possible, ABOi transplantation with desensitization is an alternative.

7. Non-HLA antibodies

The most pertinent immunologic barriers in solid organ transplantation are HLA and ABO incompatibility however; rejection episodes are reported in the absence of DSA raising the possibility of non-HLA antibodies.

Several non-HLA antibodies against epithelial and endothelial proteins are associated with poor renal graft outcomes [79]. Angiotensin II type I receptor antibodies have attracted much attention [80]. Non-HLA antibodies are not part of the immunologic risk assessment currently however; they are worth consideration in some instances.

8. Outcomes of desensitization in cardiac and lung transplantation

Desensitization protocols in cardiac and lung transplantation are based on experience from renal transplantation. As in renal transplantation, variability in the desensitization protocols, clinical endpoints, and antibody measurement techniques also exist in cardiac and lung transplantation [81]. Most cardiac and lung desensitization studies are small, have shorter follow-up periods, and report inconsistent results. Protocols vary between centers, but most comprise apheresis, IVIG, and rituximab combinations. Desensitization in cardiac and lung transplantation is conducted in a deceased donor setup, considering the unique characteristics of the individual patient and the nature of the organ being transplanted. Some centers commence desensitization before transplantation, while others administer it in the perioperative period. Below is a brief account of a few pertinent studies.

In a case-control study, thirty-five sensitized (PRA > 10%) cardiac transplant candidates were desensitized with five sessions of PE (1.5 plasma volume) and 20-gram IVIG administered after every PE. All patients underwent cardiac transplantation. Seventeen had positive CDCXM before desensitization. Negative crossmatch was achieved in seven cases. Both class I and class II DSA declined significantly post-treatment. Survival was better than the control group; however, more rejections were observed in the intervention group [81].

In another study (n=16), sensitized cardiac transplant candidates (PRA >10%) were treated with a single session of PE (1.5 plasma volume with albumin + four units FFP replacement) and 20-gram IVIG followed by triple maintenance immunosuppression regimen [82]. PRA declined from 55.5 to 34.9%. Survival and rejection rates at 22 months were similar among the intervention and control groups.

In a large observational study, 21 sensitized (PRA > 10%) cardiac transplant candidates were desensitized with plasma exchange, 2 g/kg IVIG, and rituximab (375 mg/kg^2 in refractory cases) [83]. Mean PRA declined from 70.5 to 30.2% post-desensitization. Five-year survival was 71.4% in the desensitized group compared to 81.1% in the untreated sensitized and 75.7% in the unsensitized group. ABMR rates were higher in the desensitized group (66.7%, 89.2% and 96.5%, respectively). Vasculopathy rates were similar between the groups.

In a small study, 16 sensitized left ventricular assist device (LVAD) recipients were treated with IVIG and a single dose of cyclophosphamide. Class I HLA DSA declined by 33%, but the DSA reappeared at four weeks [84]. In another study, a weekly 500 mg /kg IVIG dose reduced PRA in three LVAD recipients to 23% at one month and 52% at two months [85].

Eighteen highly sensitized lung transplant candidates (PRA ≥ 80%) were desensitized with methylprednisolone, bortezomib, rituximab, IVIG, and PE [86]. Nine patients were transplanted; two were on the waiting list at the time of publication, while seven patients were removed from the waiting list due to medical reasons. This protocol failed to reduce pretransplant PRA.

Another retrospective study desensitized fifty-three lung transplant candidates in the perioperative period with PE, IVIG, and anti-thymocyte globulin [87]. The sensitized cohort had preformed DSA, but only five had positive CDCXM. Clinical outcomes were like the unsensitized cohort.

9. Conclusion

Highly sensitized patients face longer waiting times on the transplant list than unsensitized patients. They experience greater morbidity and mortality. Sensitized patients have limited access to compatible organs. There is an unmet medical need to expand their access to transplantation.

Efforts have been made to circumvent incompatible transplants in sensitized patients, e.g., utilizing potential living donors, increasing the chances of well-matched organs *via* priority points in the regular allocation, acceptable match program, and kidney-paired donation. Although successful to a certain extent, such measures have failed to provide compatible organs to all sensitized patients. Desensitization could facilitate access to transplantation in selected sensitized patients who fail to access compatible organs.

It is worth noting that the outcomes of desensitization are inferior to compatible transplants. However, compared to dialysis, incompatible transplantation is cost-effective, enhances quality of life, and confers survival benefit. Acute and chronic ABMR risk is high in incompatible transplantation and is a significant cause of allograft loss. Infections and malignancies are frequent due to higher cumulative doses of immunosuppressive drugs.

Implementing novel and innovative strategies to avoid crossing the immunological barriers is vital. Transplantation tolerance has the potential to minimize sensitization. HLA epitope matching is a step forward in lowering post-transplant sensitization. Newer biomarkers are needed for immune monitoring and early diagnosis of graft rejection. Running multiple desensitization randomized trials is not feasible due to limited resources and finite eligible patients. Innovative trial designs such as master protocols could offer testing multiple therapeutics in one trial, thus accelerating the development of effective protocols and therapies. Moreover, standardizing HLA antibody and cPRA measurements will be a significant achievement in this field.

Acknowledgements

This work is not funded.

Conflict of interest

"The authors declare no conflict of interest."

Notes/thanks/other declarations

My parents (Muhammad Jamil and Ismat Begum), my wife, and my children supported me in completing this work. I would also acknowledge the support of my supervisors, Dr. Matthew Howes and Ida Ryland.

Author details

Asad Ullah* and Khalid AlMeshari
King Faisal Specialist Hospital, Riyadh, Saudi Arabia

*Address all correspondence to: drasadullah99@hotmail.com

References

[1] Holt DB, Lublin DM, Phelan DL, Boslaugh SE, Gandhi SK, Huddleston CB, et al. Mortality and morbidity in pre-sensitized pediatric heart transplant recipients with a positive donor crossmatch utilizing peri-operative plasmapheresis and cytolytic therapy. The Journal of Heart and Lung Transplantation. 2007;**26**(9):876-882

[2] Marfo K, Lu A, Ling M, Akalin E. Desensitization protocols and their outcome. Clinical Journal of the American Society of Nephrology. 2011;**6**(4):922-936

[3] Jordan SC, Choi J, Vo A. Kidney transplantation in highly sensitized patients. British Medical Bulletin. 2015;**114**(1):113-125

[4] Schinstock CA, Smith BH, Montgomery RA, Jordan SC, Bentall AJ, Mai M, et al. Managing highly sensitized renal transplant candidates in the era of kidney paired donation and the new kidney allocation system: Is there still a role for desensitization? Clinical Transplantation. 2019;**33**(12):e13751

[5] Shiina T, Inoko H, Kulski JK. An update of the HLA genomic region, locus information and disease associations: 2004. Tissue Antigens. 2004;**64**(6):631-649

[6] HLA alleles. 2023. Available from: https://hla.alleles.org/alleles/index.html.

[7] Klein J, Sato A. The HLA system. First of two parts. The New England Journal of Medicine. 2000;**343**(10):702-709

[8] Rose ML, Coles MI, Griffin RJ, Pomerance A, Yacoub MH. Expression of class I and class II major histocompatibility antigens in normal and transplanted human heart. Transplantation. 1986;**41**(6):776-780

[9] Lopes D, Barra T, Malheiro J, Tafulo S, Martins L, Almeida M, et al. Effect of different sensitization events on HLA alloimmunization in kidney transplantation candidates. Transplantation Proceedings. 2015;**47**(4):894-897

[10] Hyun J, Park KD, Yoo Y, Lee B, Han BY, Song EY, et al. Effects of different sensitization events on HLA alloimmunization in solid organ transplantation patients. Transplantation Proceedings. 2012;**44**(1):222-225

[11] Locke JE, Zachary AA, Warren DS, Segev DL, Houp JA, Montgomery RA, et al. Proinflammatory events are associated with significant increases in breadth and strength of HLA-specific antibody. American Journal of Transplantation. 2009;**9**(9):2136-2139

[12] Halloran PF, Schlaut J, Solez K, Srinivasa NS. The significance of the anti-class I response. II. Clinical and pathologic features of renal transplants with anti-class I-like antibody. Transplantation. 1992;**53**(3):550-555

[13] Snyder LD, Wang Z, Chen DF, Reinsmoen NL, Finlen-Copeland CA, Davis WA, et al. Implications for human leukocyte antigen antibodies after lung transplantation: A 10-year experience in 441 patients. Chest. 2013;**144**(1):226-233

[14] Reed EF, Rao P, Zhang Z, Gebel H, Bray RA, Guleria I, et al. Comprehensive assessment and standardization of solid phase multiplex-bead arrays for the detection of antibodies to HLA. American Journal of Transplantation. 2013;**13**(7):1859-1870

[15] Visentin J, Vigata M, Daburon S, Contin-Bordes C, Fremeaux-Bacchi V, Dromer C, et al. Deciphering

complement interference in anti-human leukocyte antigen antibody detection with flow beads assays. Transplantation. 2014;**98**(6):625-631

[16] Schnaidt M, Weinstock C, Jurisic M, Schmid-Horch B, Ender A, Wernet D. HLA antibody specification using single-antigen beads--a technical solution for the prozone effect. Transplantation. 2011;**92**(5):510-515

[17] Konvalinka A, Tinckam K. Utility of HLA antibody testing in kidney transplantation. Journal of the American Society of Nephrology. 2015;**26**(7):1489-1502

[18] Tinckam K. Histocompatibility methods. Transplantation Reviews (Orlando, Fla.). 2009;**23**(2):80-93

[19] Zangwill SD, Ellis TM, Zlotocha J, Jaquiss RD, Tweddell JS, Mussatto KA, et al. The virtual crossmatch--a screening tool for sensitized pediatric heart transplant recipients. Pediatric Transplantation. 2006;**10**(1):38-41

[20] Nikaein A, Cherikh W, Nelson K, Baker T, Leffell S, Bow L, et al. Organ procurement and transplantation network/united network for organ sharing histocompatibility committee collaborative study to evaluate prediction of crossmatch results in highly sensitized patients. Transplantation. 2009;**87**(4):557-562

[21] Bielmann D, Hönger G, Lutz D, Mihatsch MJ, Steiger J, Schaub S. Pretransplant risk assessment in renal allograft recipients using virtual crossmatching. American Journal of Transplantation. 2007;**7**(3):626-632

[22] Manook M, Koeser L, Ahmed Z, Robb M, Johnson R, Shaw O, et al. Post-listing survival for highly sensitised patients on the UK kidney transplant waiting list: A matched cohort analysis. Lancet. 2017;**389**(10070):727-734

[23] Noble J, Metzger A, Daligault M, Chevallier E, Bugnazet M, Bardy B, et al. Immortal time-bias-corrected survival of highly sensitized patients and HLA-desensitized kidney transplant recipients. Kidney International Reports. 2021;**6**(10):2629-2638

[24] Toyoda M, Shin BH, Ge S, Mirocha J, Thomas D, Chu M, et al. Impact of desensitization on antiviral immunity in HLA-sensitized kidney transplant recipients. Journal of Immunology Research. 2017;**2017**:5672523

[25] Kahwaji J, Sinha A, Toyoda M, Ge S, Reinsmoen N, Cao K, et al. Infectious complications in kidney-transplant recipients desensitized with rituximab and intravenous immunoglobulin. Clinical Journal of the American Society of Nephrology. 2011;**6**(12):2894-2900

[26] Ko EJ, Yu JH, Yang CW, Chung BH. Clinical outcomes of ABO- and HLA-incompatible kidney transplantation: A nationwide cohort study. Transplant International. 2017;**30**(12):1215-1225

[27] Opelz G, Morath C, Süsal C, Tran TH, Zeier M, Döhler B. Three-year outcomes following 1420 ABO-incompatible living-donor kidney transplants performed after ABO antibody reduction: Results from 101 centers. Transplantation. 2015;**99**(2):400-404

[28] Axelrod D, Lentine KL, Schnitzler MA, Luo X, Xiao H, Orandi BJ, et al. The incremental cost of incompatible living donor kidney transplantation: A National Cohort Analysis. American Journal of Transplantation. 2017;**17**(12):3123-3130

[29] Jordan SC, Ammerman N, Vo A. Implications of fc neonatal receptor (FcRn) manipulations for transplant immunotherapeutics. Transplantation. 2020;**104**(1):17-23

[30] Kahwaji J, Barker E, Pepkowitz S, Klapper E, Villicana R, Peng A, et al. Acute hemolysis after high-dose intravenous immunoglobulin therapy in highly HLA sensitized patients. Clinical Journal of the American Society of Nephrology. 2009;**4**(12):1993-1997

[31] Morath C, Becker LE, Leo A, Beimler J, Klein K, Seckinger J, et al. ABO-incompatible kidney transplantation enabled by non-antigen-specific immunoadsorption. Transplantation. 2012;**93**(8):827-834

[32] Cen SY, Branch DR. Isoagglutinin-reduced immunoglobulin retains efficacy in mouse models of immune thrombocytopenia and rheumatoid arthritis and is less likely to cause intravenous immunoglobulin-associated hemolysis. Transfusion. 2020;**60**(2):250-255

[33] Glotz D, Antoine C, Julia P, Suberbielle-Boissel C, Boudjeltia S, Fraoui R, et al. Desensitization and subsequent kidney transplantation of patients using intravenous immunoglobulins (IVIg). American Journal of Transplantation. 2002;**2**(8):758-760

[34] Jordan SC, Vo A, Bunnapradist S, Toyoda M, Peng A, Puliyanda D, et al. Intravenous immune globulin treatment inhibits crossmatch positivity and allows for successful transplantation of incompatible organs in living-donor and cadaver recipients. Transplantation. 2003;**76**(4):631-636

[35] Vo AA, Toyoda M, Peng A, Bunnapradist S, Lukovsky M, Jordan SC. Effect of induction therapy protocols on transplant outcomes in crossmatch positive renal allograft recipients desensitized with IVIG. American Journal of Transplantation. 2006;**6**(10):2384-2390

[36] Motter JD, Jackson KR, Long JJ, Waldram MM, Orandi BJ, Montgomery RA, et al. Delayed graft function and acute rejection following HLA-incompatible living donor kidney transplantation. American Journal of Transplantation. 2021;**21**(4):1612-1621

[37] Vo AA, Peng A, Toyoda M, Kahwaji J, Cao K, Lai CH, et al. Use of intravenous immune globulin and rituximab for desensitization of highly HLA-sensitized patients awaiting kidney transplantation. Transplantation. 2010;**89**(9):1095-1102

[38] Vo AA, Lukovsky M, Toyoda M, Wang J, Reinsmoen NL, Lai CH, et al. Rituximab and intravenous immune globulin for desensitization during renal transplantation. The New England Journal of Medicine. 2008;**359**(3):242-251

[39] Jordan SC, Tyan D, Stablein D, McIntosh M, Rose S, Vo A, et al. Evaluation of intravenous immunoglobulin as an agent to lower allosensitization and improve transplantation in highly sensitized adult patients with end-stage renal disease: Report of the NIH IG02 trial. Journal of the American Society of Nephrology. 2004;**15**(12):3256-3262

[40] Montgomery RA, Zachary AA, Racusen LC, Leffell MS, King KE, Burdick J, et al. Plasmapheresis and intravenous immune globulin provides effective rescue therapy for refractory humoral rejection and allows kidneys to be successfully transplanted into cross-match-positive recipients. Transplantation. 2000;**70**(6):887-895

[41] Noble J, Metzger A, Naciri Bennani H, Daligault M, Masson D, Terrec F, et al. Apheresis efficacy and tolerance in the setting of HLA-incompatible kidney transplantation. Journal of Clinical Medicine. 2021;**10**(6)

[42] Lentine KL, Axelrod D, Klein C, Simpkins C, Xiao H, Schnitzler MA,

et al. Early clinical complications after ABO-incompatible live-donor kidney transplantation: A national study of Medicare-insured recipients. Transplantation. 2014;**98**(1):54-65

[43] Haririan A, Nogueira J, Kukuruga D, Schweitzer E, Hess J, Gurk-Turner C, et al. Positive cross-match living donor kidney transplantation: Longer-term outcomes. American Journal of Transplantation. 2009;**9**(3):536-542

[44] Stegall MD, Gloor J, Winters JL, Moore SB, Degoey S. A comparison of plasmapheresis versus high-dose IVIG desensitization in renal allograft recipients with high levels of donor specific alloantibody. American Journal of Transplantation. 2006;**6**(2):346-351

[45] Loupy A, Suberbielle-Boissel C, Zuber J, Anglicheau D, Timsit MO, Martinez F, et al. Combined posttransplant prophylactic IVIg/anti-CD 20/ plasmapheresis in kidney recipients with preformed donor-specific antibodies: A pilot study. Transplantation. 2010;**89**(11):1403-1410

[46] Niederhaus SV, Muth B, Lorentzen DF, Wai P, Pirsch JD, Samaniego-Picota M, et al. Luminex-based desensitization protocols: The University of Wisconsin initial experience. Transplantation. 2011;**92**(1):12-17

[47] Vo AA, Petrozzino J, Yeung K, Sinha A, Kahwaji J, Peng A, et al. Efficacy, outcomes, and cost-effectiveness of desensitization using IVIG and rituximab. Transplantation. 2013;**95**(6):852-858

[48] Jackson AM, Kraus ES, Orandi BJ, Segev DL, Montgomery RA, Zachary AA. A closer look at rituximab induction on HLA antibody rebound following HLA-incompatible kidney transplantation. Kidney International. 2015;**87**(2):409-416

[49] Vo AA, Choi J, Cisneros K, Reinsmoen N, Haas M, Ge S, et al. Benefits of rituximab combined with intravenous immunoglobulin for desensitization in kidney transplant recipients. Transplantation. 2014;**98**(3):312-319

[50] Redfield RR, Jordan SC, Busque S, Vincenti F, Woodle ES, Desai N, et al. Safety, pharmacokinetics, and pharmacodynamic activity of obinutuzumab, a type 2 anti-CD20 monoclonal antibody for the desensitization of candidates for renal transplant. American Journal of Transplantation. 2019;**19**(11):3035-3045

[51] Junghans RP, Anderson CL. The protection receptor for IgG catabolism is the beta2-microglobulin-containing neonatal intestinal transport receptor. Proceedings of the National Academy of Sciences of the United States of America. 1996;**93**(11):5512-5516

[52] Woodle ES, Shields AR, Ejaz NS, Sadaka B, Girnita A, Walsh RC, et al. Prospective iterative trial of proteasome inhibitor-based desensitization. American Journal of Transplantation. 2015;**15**(1):101-118

[53] Moreno Gonzales MA, Gandhi MJ, Schinstock CA, Moore NA, Smith BH, Braaten NY, et al. 32 doses of bortezomib for desensitization is not well tolerated and is associated with only modest reductions in anti-HLA antibody. Transplantation. 2017;**101**(6):1222-1227

[54] Tremblay S, Driscoll JJ, Rike-Shields A, Hildeman DA, Alloway RR, Girnita AL, et al. A prospective, iterative, adaptive trial of carfilzomib-based desensitization. American Journal of Transplantation. 2020;**20**(2):411-421

[55] Bentall A, Tyan DB, Sequeira F, Everly MJ, Gandhi MJ, Cornell LD, et al.

Antibody-mediated rejection despite inhibition of terminal complement. Transplant International. 2014;**27**(12):1235-1243

[56] Vo AA, Zeevi A, Choi J, Cisneros K, Toyoda M, Kahwaji J, et al. A phase I/II placebo-controlled trial of C1-inhibitor for prevention of antibody-mediated rejection in HLA sensitized patients. Transplantation. 2015;**99**(2):299-308

[57] Jordan SC, Lorant T, Choi J, Kjellman C, Winstedt L, Bengtsson M, et al. IgG endopeptidase in highly sensitized patients undergoing transplantation. The New England Journal of Medicine. 2017;**377**(5):442-453

[58] Jordan SC, Legendre C, Desai NM, Lorant T, Bengtsson M, Lonze BE, et al. Imlifidase desensitization in crossmatch-positive, highly sensitized kidney transplant recipients: Results of an international phase 2 trial (Highdes). Transplantation. 2021;**105**(8):1808-1817

[59] Kjellman C, Maldonado AQ, Sjöholm K, Lonze BE, Montgomery RA, Runström A, et al. Outcomes at 3 years posttransplant in imlifidase-desensitized kidney transplant patients. American Journal of Transplantation. 2021;**21**(12):3907-3918

[60] Vo AA, Huang E, Ammerman N, Toyoda M, Ge S, Haas M, et al. Clazakizumab for desensitization in highly sensitized patients awaiting transplantation. American Journal of Transplantation. 2022;**22**(4):1133-1144

[61] Clatworthy MR. B-cell regulation and its application to transplantation. Transplant International. 2014;**27**(2): 117-128

[62] Bath NM, Ding X, Verhoven BM, Wilson NA, Coons L, Sukhwal A, et al. Autoantibody production significantly decreased with APRIL/BLyS blockade in murine chronic rejection kidney transplant model. PLoS One. 2019;**14**(10):e0223889

[63] Wilson NA, Bath NM, Verhoven BM, Ding X, Boldt BA, Sukhwal A, et al. APRIL/BLyS blockade reduces donor-specific antibodies in allosensitized mice. Transplantation. 2019;**103**(7):1372-1384

[64] Kwun J, Matignon M, Manook M, Guendouz S, Audard V, Kheav D, et al. Daratumumab in sensitized kidney transplantation: Potentials and limitations of experimental and clinical use. Journal of the American Society of Nephrology. 2019;**30**(7):1206-1219

[65] Hume DM, Magee JH, Kauffman HM Jr, Rittenbury MS, Prout GR Jr. Renal homotransplantation in man in modified recipients. Annals of Surgery. 1963;**158**(4):608-644

[66] Langhorst C, Ganner A, Schneider J, Prager EP, Walz G, Pisarski P, et al. Long-term follow-up of ABO-incompatible kidney transplantation in Freiburg, Germany: A single-center outcome report. Transplantation Proceedings. 2021;**53**(3):848-855

[67] Kobayashi T, Saito K. A series of surveys on assay for anti-A/B antibody by Japanese ABO-incompatible transplantation committee. Xenotransplantation. 2006;**13**(2):136-140

[68] Zhao D, Zhu L, Zhang S, Guo Z, Wang L, Pan T, et al. Case report: Successful ABO-incompatible deceased donor kidney transplantation in an infant without pre-transplant immunological treatment. Frontiers in Medicine. 2022;**9**:838738

[69] Sypek MMR, Hughes P. ABO incompatible deceased donor renal transplantation: Exploring the

possibilities. American Journal of Transplantation. 2017;**17**

[70] Tobian AA, Shirey RS, Montgomery RA, Cai W, Haas M, Ness PM, et al. ABO antibody titer and risk of antibody-mediated rejection in ABO-incompatible renal transplantation. American Journal of Transplantation. 2010;**10**(5):1247-1253

[71] Toki D, Ishida H, Setoguchi K, Shimizu T, Omoto K, Shirakawa H, et al. Acute antibody-mediated rejection in living ABO-incompatible kidney transplantation: Long-term impact and risk factors. American Journal of Transplantation. 2009;**9**(3):567-577

[72] Ishida H, Koyama I, Sawada T, Utsumi K, Murakami T, Sannomiya A, et al. Anti-AB titer changes in patients with ABO incompatibility after living related kidney transplantations: Survey of 101 cases to determine whether splenectomies are necessary for successful transplantation. Transplantation. 2000;**70**(4):681-685

[73] Masterson R, Hughes P, Walker RG, Hogan C, Haeusler M, Robertson AR, et al. ABO incompatible renal transplantation without antibody removal using conventional immunosuppression alone. American Journal of Transplantation. 2014;**14**(12):2807-2813

[74] Fuchinoue S, Ishii Y, Sawada T, Murakami T, Iwadoh K, Sannomiya A, et al. The 5-year outcome of ABO-incompatible kidney transplantation with rituximab induction. Transplantation. 2011;**91**(8):853-857

[75] Macklin PS, Morris PJ, Knight SR. A systematic review of the use of rituximab for desensitization in renal transplantation. Transplantation. 2014;**98**(8):794-805

[76] Segev DL, Simpkins CE, Warren DS, King KE, Shirey RS, Maley WR, et al. ABO incompatible high-titer renal transplantation without splenectomy or anti-CD20 treatment. American Journal of Transplantation. 2005;**5**(10):2570-2575

[77] Scurt FG, Ewert L, Mertens PR, Haller H, Schmidt BMW, Chatzikyrkou C. Clinical outcomes after ABO-incompatible renal transplantation: A systematic review and meta-analysis. Lancet. 2019;**393**(10185):2059-2072

[78] Axelrod D, Segev DL, Xiao H, Schnitzler MA, Brennan DC, Dharnidharka VR, et al. Economic impacts of ABO-incompatible live donor kidney transplantation: A national study of medicare-insured recipients. American Journal of Transplantation. 2016;**16**(5):1465-1473

[79] Sorohan BM, Baston C, Tacu D, Bucșa C, Țincu C, Vizireanu P, et al. Non-HLA antibodies in kidney transplantation: Immunity and genetic insights. Biomedicine. 2022;**10**(7)

[80] Lefaucheur C, Louis K, Philippe A, Loupy A, Coates PT. The emerging field of non-human leukocyte antigen antibodies in transplant medicine and beyond. Kidney International. 2021;**100**(4):787-798

[81] Chih S, Patel J. Desensitization strategies in adult heart transplantation-will persistence pay off? The Journal of Heart and Lung Transplantation. 2016;**35**(8):962-972

[82] Pisani BA, Mullen GM, Malinowska K, Lawless CE, Mendez J, Silver MA, et al. Plasmapheresis with intravenous immunoglobulin G is effective in patients with elevated panel reactive antibody prior to cardiac transplantation. The Journal of Heart and Lung Transplantation. 1999;**18**(7):701-706

[83] Kobashigawa JA, Patel JK, Kittleson MM, Kawano MA, Kiyosaki KK, Davis SN, et al. The long-term outcome of treated sensitized patients who undergo heart transplantation. Clinical Transplantation. 2011;**25**(1):E61-E67

[84] John R, Lietz K, Burke E, Ankersmit J, Mancini D, Suciu-Foca N, et al. Intravenous immunoglobulin reduces anti-HLA alloreactivity and shortens waiting time to cardiac transplantation in highly sensitized left ventricular assist device recipients. Circulation. 1999;**100** (19 Suppl):Ii229-Ii235

[85] Dowling RD, Jones JW, Carroll MS, Gray LA, Jr. Use of intravenous immunoglobulin in sensitized LVAD recipients. Transplantation Proceedings 1998;**30**(4):1110-1.

[86] Snyder LD, Gray AL, Reynolds JM, Arepally GM, Bedoya A, Hartwig MG, et al. Antibody desensitization therapy in highly sensitized lung transplant candidates. American Journal of Transplantation. 2014;**14**(4):849-856

[87] Tinckam KJ, Keshavjee S, Chaparro C, Barth D, Azad S, Binnie M, et al. Survival in sensitized lung transplant recipients with perioperative desensitization. American Journal of Transplantation. 2015;**15**(2):417-426

Section 2

Tissue Allograft

Chapter 4

Contemporary Approach with Mitral Valve Allograft in the Treatment of Tricuspid Valve Pathology

Mikhail D. Nuzhdin, Roman N. Komarov and Vladimir A. Bolsunovsky

Abstract

Symptomatic tricuspid valve diseases are associated with a high risk of heart failure and poor prognosis. The current valve substitutes still carry the risk of associated complications. Allografts have been considered a valuable surgical option for decades since the first reports were introduced. The challenging surgical technique along with controversial results and homograft shortage discourage surgical society from wider use of allografts in tricuspid surgery. The largest world surgical experience with mitral allograft in the treatment of tricuspid valve disease is described in the study. A total of 20 patients underwent tricuspid valve replacement by mitral homograft in two clinics from October 2021 to February 2023. Surgical technique and initial results are presented in the chapter. There was no early mortality, postoperative bleeding, myocardium infarction, stroke, or sternal wound infection. Two patients needed permanent pacemaker implantation after redoing surgery before discharge. In the follow-up period, two patients suffered from a relapse of infective endocarditis in 3 and 6 months postoperatively with moderate homograft dysfunction, none of them underwent reintervention. There was no late mortality or permanent pacemaker implantation in the follow-up period. Satisfactory clinical and hemodynamic results, reproduceable technique and accessibility make homografts plausible valve substitutes in tricuspid surgery.

Keywords: allograft, mitral valve, tricuspid valve, endocarditis, valve prosthesis

1. Introduction

The prevalence of moderate-to-severe tricuspid regurgitation (TR) increases with age, affecting about 4% of the patients aged 75 years and is observed in up to 0.6% of the general population [1].

Primary TR usually appears as a result of infective endocarditis, rheumatic heart disease, carcinoid syndrome, myxomatous disease, endomyocardial fibrosis, congenital heart disease, and other less frequent causes, such as thoracic trauma and iatrogenic damage [2].

Severe TR is associated with poor survival and worsening heart failure symptoms [1, 3–5].

The choice between a biological valve and a mechanical valve for the tricuspid position is still controversial [6].

The use of allograft substitutes or autografts is not uniform across European and American units and is greatly dependent on surgeons' individual experience and training [7].

Technical challenge and the lack of training in these techniques over the last 10 years, coupled with the absence of readily available homograft valves at many centers, has restricted the widespread use of this substitute, confining the "art" of homograft surgery to the hands of a small group of surgeons [8].

It is undeniable that when such factors as the severity of the destructive process or its extension to the valves are involved, the balance in the choice of the most suitable substitute is critically weighted toward homografts over conventional stented or mechanical prostheses [7].

Replacement of the tricuspid valve (TVR) using a homograft could provide favorable in-hospital and mid- to long-term clinical outcomes for patients with a variety of causes and age groups, despite slightly complex surgical technique compared with prosthetic valve replacement. This procedure might be useful, particularly in treating active bacterial endocarditis or young patients, in centers at which homograft tissue is available [9].

2. Current clinical guidelines on the management of tricuspid valve diseases

In spite of clinical significance of early surgery, TV interventions are often initiated too late [10, 11]. Appropriate timing of tricuspid surgery is essential to avoid irreversible right ventricle (RV) dysfunction with subsequent increased surgical risk [12, 13]. Not only have clinical and diagnostic thresholds been defined but also there is inconclusive data for prognostic value of tricuspid annular pulmonary systolic excursion in patients with primary TR undergoing surgical intervention. Clinical importance of tricuspid annulus plane systolic excursion (TAPSE) and RV reverse remodeling have been highlighted predominantly in secondary tricuspid valve regurgitation studies [14, 15].

2.1 Indication for tricuspid valve intervention and prosthesis choice

Regarding severe primary TR, recent guidelines recommend surgical intervention in symptomatic patients. In selected asymptomatic or mildly symptomatic patients who are appropriate for surgery, an intervention should also be considered when RV dilatation or declining RV function is observed.

Whenever possible, annuloplasty with prosthetic rings is preferable to valve replacement, which should only be considered when the tricuspid valve leaflets are tethered and the annulus severely dilated [14, 16]. In the presence of a cardiac implantable electronic device lead, the technique used should be adapted to the patient's condition and the surgeon's experience [17].

TVR procedure accounts for less than 10% of all interventions on the tricuspid valve [18, 19].

Replacement of the tricuspid valve is a necessary measure in cases where annuloplasty is not possible (infective endocarditis, Ebstein's anomaly, reoperation after unsuccessful plastic surgery, prosthetic endocarditis) [19].

Mechanical valves are considered better durability, but higher risk of thrombosis, bleeding complication due to anticoagulation and decreased turbulence [19–21].

Biological prostheses do not require long-term anticoagulants and have a lower risk of hemorrhagic events, but at the same time durability is limited as a result of structural valve deterioration [16].

There are no specific guidelines devoted to a type of prosthetic valve that would be the best choice in the tricuspid position [22].

One meta-analysis strongly indicates the risk of thrombosis in mechanical valves is higher, while other end-points are not significantly different between the two types of valves [6].

Transcatheter tricuspid valve interventions may be considered by the Heart Team at experienced Heart Valve Centers in symptomatic, inoperable, and anatomically eligible patients in whom symptomatic or prognostic improvement can be expected. For detailed anatomical evaluation, transesophageal (TOE) echocardiography (ECHO) and cardiac computed tomography may be preferred owing to higher spatial resolution [23, 24].

3. Historical insight on allograft valve substitutes for tricuspid valve surgery

The first mitral homograft in humans was performed in 1965 by Senning. Since that time, there has been a limited number of implants mainly because of technical difficulties related to the insertion of the papillary muscles. Homologous transplantation of the mitral valve was also applied for TVR in the case of infective endocarditis or for the replacement of a degenerated bioprosthesis. Satisfactory results have been reported. However, due to the lack of anatomical landmarks, the implantation procedure has remained technically challenging. Thus until further progress demonstrated a clear superiority of the mitral homograft, bioprosthesis has remained the gold standard for replacing the mitral or the tricuspid valve with a biological substitute [25].

The most significant surgical experience with allografts in tricuspid surgery was reported by Hvass U., et al., 2002–9 patients, Couetil J.-P.A., 2002–7 patients, Kalangos A., 2004–8 patients [26–28].

The largest world experience with tricuspid homografts in the tricuspid position was depicted by Shrestha B.M.S. in 2010 and included 14 patients [9].

It should be mentioned that the overall allografts data regarding both mitral and tricuspid valve surgery is confined to small case series with a lack of initial and long-term results. Surgical techniques have not been described properly as well.

3.1 Indication for surgery and types of allografts used in tricuspid position

According to world surgical experience of allografts for tricuspid valve disease, the most relevant indications for interventions were: infective endocarditis, rheumatic heart disease, degenerative and congenital heart diseases including Ebshtein anomaly, bioprosthetic dysfunction (**Table 1**) [9, 29, 30]. Allografts had been utilized both in primary and redo cases [9, 29].

3.2 Surgical techniques

Historically, mitral and tricuspid homografts in the tricuspid position were used either for total (complete) valve replacement or for partial TVR, usually anterior tricuspid leaflet. Positioning of the mitral homograft in the tricuspid annulus also varied throughout the studies. Anti-anatomical orientation of the mitral homograft (anterior homograft leaflet to the septal portion of tricuspid annulus) was first introduced by J.L.Pomar, C.A.Mesters and many other authors followed such technique (**Table 2**) [30]. Conversely, anatomical orientation (anterior homograft leaflet to anterior portion of tricuspid annulus) was proposed only by Couetil J.-P.A., 2002 and Kalangos A., 2004 [27, 28].

The most challenging issue has always been securing homograft's papillary muscles in the right ventricle cavity. Right ventricle papillary muscles, along with the free wall and interventricular septum had been proposed for papillary muscle fixation (**Table 2**). Annuloplasty as a bail-out procedure was described in some studies, by the way, the data is inconclusive.

3.3 Outcomes

Initial and long-term results of allografts in tricuspid surgery are summarized in **Table 3**. Early and 30-day mortality was not reported in any study. Postoperative complications included a complete atrioventricular block in one study from Ostrovsky Y., 2015 and – postoperative bleeding that required resternotomy in another study from Luciani G.B., 2021 [32, 33]. Overall survival at the end of the follow-up period was 100 [90,7–100] %, freedom from graft dysfunction — 100%, and freedom from reoperation — 100 [79–100] %. All authors confirmed complete recovery from infection in patients who had undergone surgery due to infective endocarditis.

	Author, year	N	Etiology	Allograft type
1	Di Summa et al., [29]	1	Infective endocarditis	Tricuspid
2	Pomar and Mesters [30]	3	Infective endocarditis	Mitral
3	Miyagishima [31]	5	Infective endocarditis	Mitral
4	Hvass [26]	9	Infective endocarditis, congenital	Mitral
5	Couetil [27]	7	Infective endocarditis	Mitral
6	Kalangos [28]	8	Failed tricuspid repair in children	Mitral
7	Shrestha [9]	14	Infective endocarditis, congenital and rheumatic heart disease, redo surgery	Tricuspid (n = 13)
8	Ostrovsky [32]	2	Infective endocarditis	Mitral
9	Luciani [33]	1	Infective endocarditis	Pulmonary

Table 1.
Indication for surgery and allograft type for tricuspid valve (world data).

	Author, year	N	Graft orientation	Completeness of repair	Papillary muscle fixation	Annuloplasty
1	Di Summa et al., [29]	1	N/d	Total	RV papillary muscles	—
2	Pomar and Mesters [30]	3	Anti-anatomical	Total	RV free wall	N/d
3	Miyagishima et al. [31]	5	Anti-anatomical	Total	RV free wall	Rigid mitral ring
4	Hvass et al. [26]	9	Anti-anatomical	Total	RV free wall	Flexible annuloplasty ring
5	Couetil [27]	7	Anatomical	Partial	RV free wall	Ring
6	Kalangos [28]	8	Anatomical	Total	IVS RV free wall	Ring
7	Shrestha [9]	14	Anatomical	Partial	RV papillary muscles IVS RV free wall	Ring (n = 5), Suture annuloplasty (n = 2)
8	Ostrovsky [32]	2	Anti-anatomical	Total	IVS RV free wall	—
9	Luciani [33]	1	N/a	Total	RV papillary muscles	—

N – number of patients; N/d – no data available; RV – right ventricle; IVS – Interventricular septum.

Table 2.
Surgical aspects for homograft tricuspid valve replacement (world experience).

4. Contemporary approach for mitral allograft as a feasible prosthetic substitute in tricuspid valve surgery. Two-center experience

4.1 Patients and methods

4.1.1 Patient's population

Between October 2021 and February 2023, a total of 20 patients underwent TVR by means of mitral homograft at the two institutions ("Chelyabinsk Regional Clinical Hospital" and the "Sechenov University"). This study was approved by the Regional Ethics Committee of the 2 hospitals, and all patients signed their informed consent. The Institutional Review Board approved this study (# 19_2021) on 18 October 2021. The baseline clinical characteristic is depicted in **Table 4**.

4.1.2 Preoperative assessment and indication for surgery

Preoperative assessment included calculating EuroScore II risk, Tri-Score band, and MELD Score regarding the patient's age, clinical symptoms of right heart failure, ejection fraction, daily Furosemide intake, and major laboratory findings. Estimated and predicted in-hospital mortality and morbidity along with 3-month predicted mortality were taken into consideration [34–36].

	Author, year	N	Follow-up, month	Early and 30-day mortality	Survival	Freedom from graft dysfunction	Reoperation freedom
1	Di Summa et al. [29]	1	6	0	100%		100%
2	Pomar and Mesters [30]	3	252	0	33%		33%
3	Miyagishima et al. [31]	5	12	0	80%	N/d	N/d
4	Hvass et al. [26]	9	3	0	100%	100%	100%
5	Couetil [27]	7	46	0	85,8%	N/d	100%
6	Kalangos [28]	8	68	0	100%	100%	100%
7	Shrestha [9], 2010	14	126	0	100%	100%	78,6%
8	Ostrovsky [32], 2015	2	3	0	100%	100%	100%
9	Luciani [33], 2021	1	18	0	100%	100%	100%

N – number of patients; N/d – no data available.

Table 3.
Early and long-term outcomes for homograft tricuspid valve replacement (world experience).

4.1.3 Surgical intervention

TVR was performed using conventional cardiopulmonary bypass with bicaval cannulation and either cold blood or crystalloid cardioplegia infusion under the full-sternotomy.

4.2 Surgical technique for tricuspid valve replacement by means of mitral homograft

Homograft delivery was carried out by means of express airlines as soon as the decision to use homograft as a valve substitute had been made. All homografts were ordered from Saint-Petersburg Homograft Bank. Homografts implanted in patients were produced according to the specifications TU 9398-001-80,966,705. The starting material for the manufacture of homografts is the tissue components of the cardiovascular system of a deceased person. Unlike other similar methods of preservation, a sparing technique of osmolar decellularization and preservation of the native structure of the connective tissue matrix has been used. The manufacturing technology of this medical product ensures maximum preservation of the native properties of the connective tissue matrix and high hemocompatibility.

Important features of these products are their elasticity and plasticity, which makes it easy to model products during their implantation, taking into account the

Baseline characteristics	n (n = 20)
Age (years), mean ± SD	38,8 ± 10,7
Height (cм), mean ± SD	170,6 ± 7,43
Body mass index (kg/m^2), mean ± SD	23,6 ± 3,26
Body surface area (m^2), mean ± SD	1,81 ± 0,14
Weight (kg), mean ± SD	69,3 ± 10,1
EuroScore II, %, Me [Q1-Q3]	2 [1,3-2,5]
MELD Score, Me [Q1-Q3]	8 [7–9]
Estimated_3d_mortality, Me [Q1-Q3]	1,9 [1,9-1,9]
Tri-Score, Me [Q1-Q3]	4 [4–6]
Predicted in-hospital mortality(%), Me [Q1-Q3]	8[8–22]
Total bilirubin, Me [Q1-Q3]	14,8 [7,35-23,1]
Total protein, M ± SD	76,7 ± 8,69
Albumin, M ± SD	40,1 ± 6,63
Creatinin (mcmol/l), Me [Q1-Q3]	83 [74,8-95,5]
Daily dose furosemide (mg/day), Me [Q1-Q3]	40 [40–80]
Clinical signs	
Dyspnea, n (%)	20 (100%)
Leg oedema, n (%)	8 (40%)
Ascites, n (%)	5 (25%)
Uncontrolled infection, n (%)	5 (25%)
NYHA class, n (%)	II - 3 (15%) III - 12 (60%) IV - 5 (25%)
Pneumonia, n (%)	5 (25%)
Positive blood culture, n (%)	3 (15%)
Hepatitis C, n (%)	11 (55%)
HIV, n (%)	5 (25%)
ARVT, n (%)	5 (25%)
Under antibiotic therapy, n (%)	6 (30%)

M ± SD – mean and standard deviation; Me [Q1-Q3] – median and interquartile range. NYHA – New York Heart Association; HIV – human immune virus; ARVT – anti-retrovirus therapy.

Table 4.
Patient characteristics.

characteristics of the patient's individual anatomy. Homografts are stored at a temperature of 0 to 4 degrees Celsius or be cryopreserved and stored at a temperature of minus 150 degrees Celsius.

A homograft for mitral valve replacement is represented by a mitral valve with a muscular layer in the area of the annulus fibrosus, a 5 mm rim of the left atrial endocardium, a chordal apparatus of the mitral valve, and a section of papillary (papillary) muscles with a sutured platform.

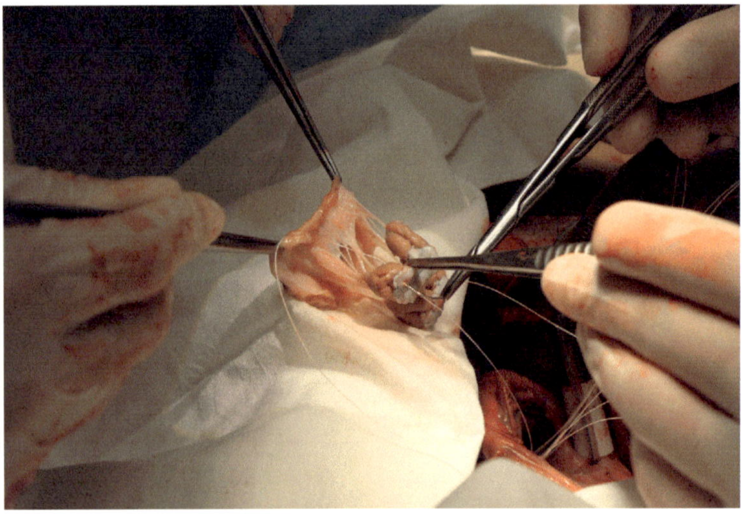

Figure 1.
Mitral homograft with papillary muscles reinforced with pericardial flap.

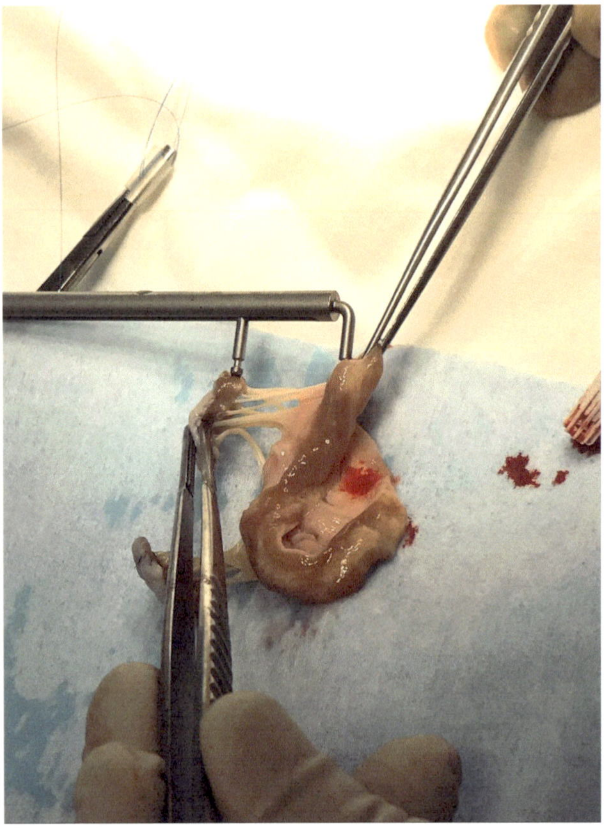

Figure 2.
Measurement of the distance between homograft annulus to the papillary muscle head.

In the manufacture of a medical product, the distance of the marginal chords to the papillary area is estimated and taken into account during its formation.

Freshly prepared products are stored in solution for 3 months. During this period should be implanted.

The sterility of each product is confirmed by negative microbiological and virological tests. It should be mentioned that the base of each homograft papillary muscle is reinforced with a pericardial flap for reliable suturing (**Figure 1**).

Assuming there is no guideline for sizing homografts preoperatively, our choice was based on measured tricuspid annulus diameter and surgical experience. The patient's body size, right ventricle dimensions, and pulmonary artery pressure were taken into account as well.

The original technique for TVR with mitral homograft that was proposed and utilized in our clinical had been described previously [37]. Further steps were partially modified in order to simplify the procedure and make results more predictable and stable. Those were: 1. keeping mitral homograft posterior leaflet totally oriented to septal portion of tricuspid annulus and anterior mitral homograft leaflet oriented straight opposite to the septal part, which is believed to preserve natural orientation of all homograft structures as a functional unit; 2. Harvesting and taking away any residual muscular tissue of homograft annulus; 3. Systematic use of rigid ring, either synthetic or biological (bovine pericardium); 4. Correction of any residual leaflet prolapse by suturing polytetrafluoroethylene (PTFE) chords. We did not take into account the complex anatomy of papillary muscle and diverse papillary head distribution, whereas the number of main muscles (generally 2), and their size was given full respect. Homograft papillary muscles were pre-implanted first in order to reduce the risk of tear of interventricular myocardium when the annulus was in place. The proper point for papillaries was chosen in accordance with measurements made on homograft (**Figures 2** and **3**).

In all cases, homograft papillary muscles were reimplanted to the interventricular septum just above the reflection of the supraventricular crest of the RV (for anterolateral homograft papillary muscle) and left to the anterior papillary muscle of the RV (for posteromedial homograft muscle) (**Figure 3**). Interpapillary distance was measured in all cases as well in order not to distort homograft anatomy (**Figure 4**). For papillary muscle, fixation were routinely used PTFE chords. Not only did it provide firm fixation, but also allowed further leaflet repair in case of residual prolapse (**Figure 5**).

Based on these principles, mitral homograft was oriented as a functional unit in the inlet part of the right ventricle cavity, given full respect to mitral valve apparatus and RV hemodynamic. Never have we ever considered the RV-free wall for papillary muscle fixation.

4.2.1 Echocardiographic assessment

Transthoracic ECHO was routinely performed by experienced medical technologists, before surgery, at 1 week, 6 months, and 1 year postoperatively. Preoperative and postoperative assessments, including grading of valve regurgitation, ventricles volumes, and function, were obtained according to guidelines [38]. All patients underwent intrapreoperative TOE ECHO to determine the degree of severity and location of tricuspid regurgitation and the final repair result.

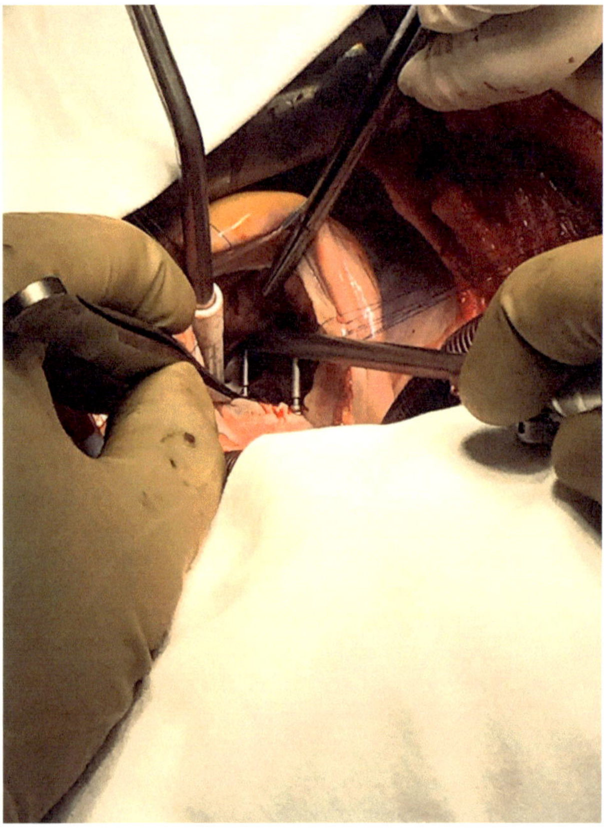

Figure 3.
Measurement of the distance between tricuspid annulus to the septum (just above the supraventricular crest).

4.2.2 Follow-up

Follow-up data after the operation were obtained through a review of patient medical records during follow-up visits and telephone interviews.

4.2.3 Definitions and data collection

Early and mid-term complications, as well as morbidity and mortality data, were summarized according to recommendations for reporting outcomes after cardiac valve interventions [39]. Early mortality was defined as in-hospital and 30-day mortality; late mortality was defined as death occurring beyond this period. Early graft dysfunction was defined as any homograft regurgitation with a vena contracta more than 0,7 cm due to central jet or periannular leak.

4.3 Statistical analysis

Descriptive statistics included continuous variables as the mean ± standard deviation or as the median and interquartile range; categorical variables are summarized as frequencies and percentages. Statistical analyses were performed using IBM SPSS Statistics Software for Windows, version 26.0 (IBM Corporation, Armonk, NY, USA).

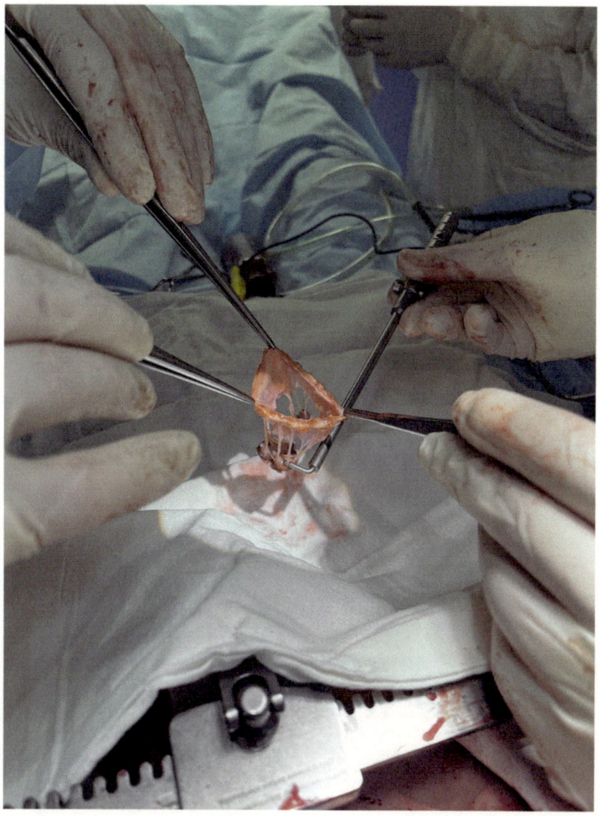

Figure 4.
Measurement of interpapillary muscle distance on the mitral homograft.

5. Results

5.1 Patient characteristics

Baseline characteristics are detailed in **Table 4**. The mean age was 38,8 ± 10,7 years, and 30% of the patients were female. All patients were operated on with acceptable predicted operative risk, in-hospital and 3-month mortality. Mean EuroScore II was 2 [1,3-2,5], while estimated 3-month mortality and predicted in-hospital mortality calculated by MELD Score and more specific Tri-Score were 1,9 [1,9-1,9] % and 8 [8–22] %, respectively. In our clinic, we persuaded the policy of early intervention rather than "watchful waiting" in terms of multiorgan failure in patients with severe tricuspid regurgitation, which is why there were no significant changes in major laboratory parameters before surgery. The mean daily dose of furosemide intake (mg/day) was 40 [40–80]. The majority of patients were highly symptomatic with III-IV NYHA class - 17 (85%). Surgical indications were based on the symptoms of heart failure in 15 (75%) patients, while the rest 5 (25%) had signs of uncontrolled infection despite appropriate antibiotic therapy. Due to prolong preoperative antibiotic medication, only 3 (15%) patients showed positive blood culture samples.

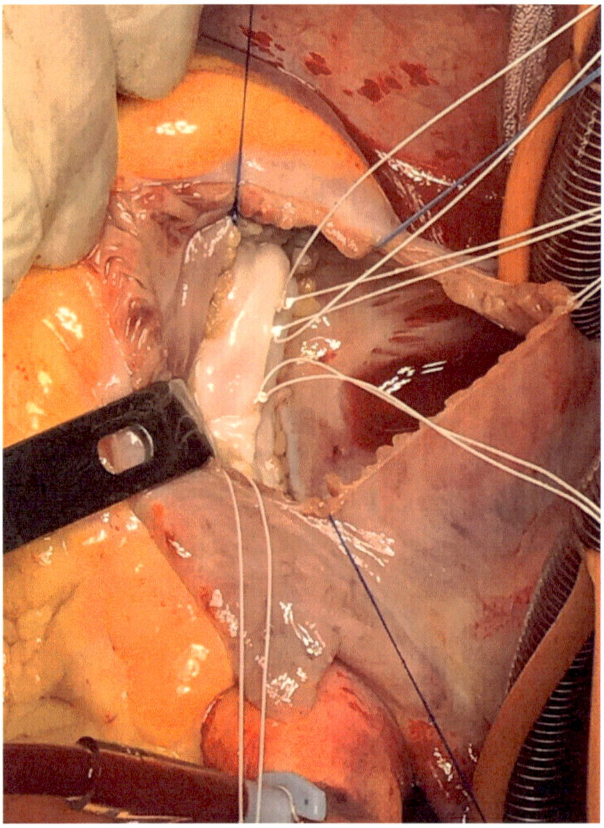

Figure 5.
PTFE chords are passed through the homograft leaflet.

5.2 Etiology of tricuspid valve disease and type of procedure

The etiology of tricuspid valve disease and types of procedures are depicted in **Table 5**. Among patients who underwent surgery, tricuspid regurgitation appeared due to infective endocarditis in 15 (75%) patients, as part of congenital disease in 4 (20%) patients, and degenerative lesions in 3 (15%) patients. Bioprosthetic failure accounted for 3 (15%) patients and mechanical prosthesis thrombosis in 1 patient. Most of the patients underwent intervention under either elective or urgent settings—8 (40%) and 10 (50%) patients respectively. Emergent tricuspid valve replacement was performed in two patients. There were 15 (75%) primary cases and 5 (25%) redo cases with a median interval from the first surgery 26 [3.5–78] months.

5.3 Early complications, mortality, and outcomes

Early postoperative complications and outcomes are highlighted in **Table 6**. There was no in-hospital mortality, postoperative myocardial infarction, stroke, renal failure, wound complications, and bleeding required resternotomy. Two patients who underwent redo surgery required permanent pacemaker implantation due to severe tricuspid annulus damage. In one patient with fungal prosthetic endocarditis, a parahomograft leak was diagnosed but did not require reoperation. This

Etiology of tricuspid valve disease	
Infective endocarditis, n (%)	15 (75%)
Degenerative, n (%)	3 (15%)
Congenital, n (%)	4 (20%)
Other, n (%)	2 (10%)
Bioprosthetic disfunction, n (%)	3 (15%)
Mechanical prosthesis thrombosis, n (%)	1 (5%)
Type of procedure	
Urgent, n (%)	10 (50%)
Emergent, n (%)	2 (10%)
Elective, n (%)	8 (40%)
Primary operation, n (%)	15 (75%)
Redo, n (%)	5 (25%)
Time from primary operation (months), Me [Q1-Q3]	26 [3,5–78]

Me [Q1-Q3] – median and interquartile range.

Table 5.
Etiology of tricuspid valve disease and type of procedure.

complication was considered as an early homograft dysfunction, nevertheless, it did not prevent a patient from complete endocarditis recovery and successful discharge from the hospital. In the follow-up period, two patients experienced a relapse of infective endocarditis in 3 and 6 months postoperatively with moderate homograft dysfunction, nevertheless, such dysfunction was tolerated well and patients recovered from infection. Patients have not been scheduled for redo operation yet. One patient had the second episode of endocarditis 1 year postoperatively and the affected valve was the aortic valve, whereas the mitral homograft was competent. There was no late mortality, or permanent pacemaker implantation in the follow-up period.

6. Discussion

Tricuspid valve operations continue to be among the most infrequently performed cardiac surgical procedures. An analysis of the Society of Thoracic Surgeons database reported only approximately 5000 tricuspid valve procedures performed per year, and most of these procedures were repairs [11].

TVR is therefore even less common, especially when it is performed in isolation [40].

It is not surprising that institutional analyses often evaluate multiple decades of operative practice to analyze fewer than 100 TVR [41]. Despite the fact that TVR has not seemed to be complicated in terms of surgical technique, operative mortality is still reported to be high, moreover, there are quite variable outcomes among studies. Leviner and colleagues reported 5.7% 30-days mortality and 14.3% 1-year mortality for the whole cohort, with a slightly higher, but not statistically significant, mortality risk for those patients who underwent isolated TVR [41]. According to Cheng Z., early mortality after TVR was 0–23.46% for biological valves and 3.03–40% for

Postoperative complications	N = 20
Myocardial infarction, n (%)	0 (0%)
Stroke, n (%)	0 (0%)
Pulmonary embolism, n (%)	0 (0%)
Pneumonia, n (%)	3 (15%)
Major bleeding, n (%)	0 (0%)
Resternotomy, n (%)	0 (0%)
Renal failure, n (%)	0 (0%)
Permanent pacemaker implantation, n (%)	2 (10%)
Other complications, n (%)	2 (10%)
Operative mortality, n (%)	0 (0%)
30-day mortality, n (%)	0 (0%)
Early graft dysfunction, n (%)	1 (5%)
PASP (mmHg), Me [Q1-Q3]	30 [30–35]
VC, Me [Q1-Q3]	0,1 [0,1-0,3]
Peak PG, Me [Q1-Q3]	5,1 [5–8]
Mean PG, M ± SD	3,16 ± 1,39

Me [Q1-Q3] – median and interquartile range; M ± SD – mean and standard deviation; PASP – pulmonary artery systolic pressure; VC – vena contracta on mitral homograft; Peak PG – peak transhomograft diastolic pressure gradient; Mean PG – mean transhomograft diastolic pressure gradient.

Table 6.
Early complications, mortality, and outcomes.

mechanical valves respectively, while the reoperation rate of biological valves was 1.94–22% while mechanical prostheses were 0.83–19.57% [6].

Regarding other significant postoperative complications, bleeding required resternotomy, and permanent pacemaker implantation remain to be unacceptably high—25.81 and 18.18% respectively, even in current reports devoted to isolated TVR with either biological or mechanical prosthesis [41]. In our study, zero mortality, and low postoperative complication rates were achieved. Having been proposed for TVR, mechanical and biological valves did not prove their complication-free profile, nevertheless, these valve substitutes are still recommended.

Among those studies that gave insight into feasibility of allografts in tricuspid surgery, there were a lot of inconclusive results in terms of surgical technique, and early- and long-term results. This fact could be explained by limited experience, homograft shortage, and low accessibility, as well as more complex surgical techniques. By the way, available data represent excellent initial results with allograft valves in the treatment of tricuspid valve disease [9, 31, 34]. Comparative studies with commonly used biological and mechanical prosthesis have not been conducted which increase the importance of our study by providing the relevant experience with mitral homografts in the tricuspid position. Obvious beneficial effects, derived from using homografts, could be a low reinfection rate, better hemodynamic performance, and no need for anticoagulation therapy, further valve repair options in case of endocarditis relapse or annular dilatation [42]. Not only does the homograft valve in tricuspid position allow further open valve repair, but also provides some opportunities for transcatheter TVR [43].

When it comes to possible drawbacks of using homografts in tricuspid surgery, such possible disadvantages are brought to mind—unpredictable long-term durability and variety of preserving methods for homograft tissue which therefore might rise or sustain existing reluctance to homograft surgery. Banking on the long-term durability of homograft tissue, relevant scientific data will be available provided a larger surgical experience appears. In accordance with Campelos P., long-term durability could generally be achieved for mitral homograft, but the data is confined to one report [30]. Recent advances in decellularized allografts for aortic valve surgery only encourage wider utilizing homograft valves in cardiac surgery [44]. The type of conduit is considered to be one of the most important factors in long-term durability, for example, the survival rate of the pulmonary conduit is higher than that of aortic conduit [45, 46]. Baltivala et al. found that the graft survival rate of patients with a history of transplantation was worse than that of other patients [47]. The relationship between bioactivity and durability of homograft valved conduit is still controversial. Fibroblasts living in the graft can reshape and reconstruct collagen structure and extracellular matrix, thus enhancing durability [48]. However, these unevenly distributed fibroblasts may have phenotypic changes and abnormal biological behavior due to immune responses or environmental changes. Decellularized valved conduits demonstrate almost complete removal of cells and cellular components by histological and immunocytochemical analysis without corresponding changes in biomechanics *in vitro* [49]. Studies compared rejection rate, immune response, and cellular activity in atrioventricular homografts vs. aortic and pulmonary homografts have not been published yet due to the complexity of comparison and different hemodynamic patterns, though it should be one of the future directions in homograft tissue science, implicated to cardio-vascular surgery.

7. Conclusion

Tricuspid valve used to be a "forgotten" valve in terms of hemodynamic consequences and appropriate time of surgery. Still, there is no ideal valve substitute for tricuspid valve replacement in cases of severe leaflet damage when valve repair is not feasible. A variety of challenging circumstances and unresolved issues exist in the treatment of tricuspid valve disease, which encourages us to find alternative solution in such clinical scenarios like active infective endocarditis, prosthetic endocarditis, and dysfunction where commonly used prosthetic material does not seem to be perfect. Assuming our initial experience with mitral homograft for tricuspid valve replacement, allograft tissue valves might take place as a plausible valve substitute, especially in patients with endocarditis, either native or prosthetic. Excellent hemodynamic performance along with highly acceptable clinical results could be achieved with mitral homografts in tricuspid surgery according to the results of our study. Low risk of perioperative complications, zero early and mid-term mortality, as well as no need for redo surgery in one postoperative year allow us to consider mitral homograft as an alternative substitute to the biological and mechanical prosthesis in tricuspid valve surgery.

Conflict of interest

The authors declare no conflict of interest.

Author details

Mikhail D. Nuzhdin[1]*, Roman N. Komarov[2] and Vladimir A. Bolsunovsky[3]

1 State Budgetary Healthcare Institution Chelyabinsk Regional Clinical Hospital, Chelyabinsk, Russian Federation

2 Federal State Autonomous Educational Institution of Higher Education First Moscow State Medical University Named After I.M. Sechenova of the Ministry of Health of the Russian Federation (Sechenov University), Moscow, Russian Federation

3 Sain-Petersburg Homograft Bank, St. Petersburg, Russian Federation

*Address all correspondence to: austesla2022@gmail.com

References

[1] Topilsky Y, Maltais S, Medina Inojosa J, Oguz D, Michelena H, Maalouf J, et al. Burden of tricuspid regurgitation in patients diagnosed in the community setting. JACC: Cardiovascular Imaging. 2019;**12**(3):433-442. DOI: 10.1016/j.jcmg.2018.06.014 Epub 2018 Aug 15

[2] Vahanian A, Beyersdorf F, Praz F, Milojevic M, Baldus S, Bauersachs J, et al. 2021 ESC/EACTS guidelines for the management of valvular heart disease: Developed by the task force for the management of valvular heart disease of the European Society of Cardiology (ESC) and the European Association for Cardio-Thoracic Surgery (EACTS). European Heart Journal. 2022;**43**(7):561-632. DOI: 10.1093/eurheartj/ehab395

[3] Benfari G, Antoine C, Miller WL, Thapa P, Topilsky Y, Rossi A, et al. Excess mortality associated with functional tricuspid regurgitation complicating heart failure with reduced ejection fraction. Circulation. 2019;**140**(3):196-206. DOI: 10.1161/CIRCULATIONAHA.118.038946 Epub 2019 May 23

[4] Chorin E, Rozenbaum Z, Topilsky Y, Konigstein M, Ziv-Baran T, Richert E, et al. Tricuspid regurgitation and long-term clinical outcomes. European Heart Journal Cardiovascular Imaging. 2020;**21**(2):157-165. DOI: 10.1093/ehjci/jez216

[5] Topilsky Y, Inojosa JM, Benfari G, Vaturi O, Maltais S, Michelena H, et al. Clinical presentation and outcome of tricuspid regurgitation in patients with systolic dysfunction. European Heart Journal. 2018;**39**(39):3584-3592. DOI: 10.1093/eurheartj/ehy434

[6] Cheng Z, Fang T, Wang D, Guo Y. Tricuspid valve replacement: Mechanical or biological prostheses? A systematic review and meta-analysis. The Heart Surgery Forum. 2021;**24**(2):E209-E214. DOI: 10.1532/hsf.3531

[7] Nappi F, Spadaccio C, Acar C. Use of allogeneic tissue to treat infective valvular disease: Has everything been said? The Journal of Thoracic and Cardiovascular Surgery. 2017;**153**(4):824-828. DOI: 10.1016/j.jtcvs.2016.09.071 Epub 2016 Oct 24

[8] Kirklin JK. Challenging homografts as the holy grail for aortic valve endocarditis. The Journal of Thoracic and Cardiovascular Surgery. 2016;**151**(5):1230-1231. DOI: 10.1016/j.jtcvs.2015.12.009 Epub 2015 Dec 13

[9] Shrestha BM, Fukushima S, Vrtik M, Chong IH, Sparks L, Jalali H, et al. Partial replacement of tricuspid valve using cryopreserved homograft. The Annals of Thoracic Surgery. 2010;**89**(4):1187-1194. DOI: 10.1016/j.athoracsur.2009.12.047

[10] Kadri AN, Menon V, Sammour YM, Gajulapalli RD, Meenakshisundaram C, Nusairat L, et al. Outcomes of patients with severe tricuspid regurgitation and congestive heart failure. Heart. 2019;**105**(23):1813-1817. DOI: 10.1136/heartjnl-2019-315004 Epub 2019 Aug 17

[11] Kilic A, Saha-Chaudhuri P, Rankin JS, Conte JV. Trends and outcomes of tricuspid valve surgery in North America: An analysis of more than 50,000 patients from the Society of Thoracic Surgeons database. The Annals of Thoracic Surgery. 2013;**96**(5):1546-1552; discussion 1552. DOI: 10.1016/j.athoracsur.2013.06.031 Epub 2013 Sep 23

[12] Dreyfus J, Ghalem N, Garbarz E, Cimadevilla C, Nataf P, Vahanian A, et al. Timing of referral of patients with severe isolated tricuspid valve regurgitation to surgeons (from a French Nationwide database). The American Journal of Cardiology. 2018;**122**(2):323-326. DOI: 10.1016/j.amjcard.2018.04.003 Epub 2018 Apr 12

[13] Antunes MJ, Rodríguez-Palomares J, Prendergast B, De Bonis M, Rosenhek R, Al-Attar N, et al. ESC working groups of cardiovascular surgery and Valvular heart disease. Management of tricuspid valve regurgitation: Position statement of the European Society of Cardiology Working Groups of cardiovascular surgery and Valvular heart disease. European Journal of Cardio-Thoracic Surgery. 2017;**52**(6):1022-1030. DOI: 10.1093/ejcts/ezx279

[14] Dreyfus GD, Corbi PJ, Chan KM, Bahrami T. Secondary tricuspid regurgitation or dilatation: Which should be the criteria for surgical repair? The Annals of Thoracic Surgery. 2005;**79**(1):127-132. DOI: 10.1016/j.athoracsur.2004.06.057

[15] Brescia AA, Ward ST, TMF W, Rosenbloom LM, Baker M, Khan S, et al. Outcomes of guideline-directed concomitant Annuloplasty for functional tricuspid regurgitation. The Annals of Thoracic Surgery. 2020;**109**(4):1227-1232. DOI: 10.1016/j.athoracsur.2019.07.035 Epub 2019 Aug 31

[16] Chang BC, Lim SH, Yi G, Hong YS, Lee S, Yoo KJ, et al. Long-term clinical results of tricuspid valve replacement. The Annals of Thoracic Surgery. 2006;**81**(4):1317-1323, discussion 1323-4. DOI: 10.1016/j.athoracsur.2005.11.005

[17] Glikson M, Nielsen JC, Kronborg MB, Michowitz Y, Auricchio A, Barbash IM, et al. 2021 ESC guidelines on cardiac pacing and cardiac resynchronization therapy. European Heart Journal. 2021;**42**(35):3427-3520. DOI: 10.1093/eurheartj/ehab364 Erratum in: Eur Heart J. 2022 May 1;43(17):1651

[18] Ratnatunga CP, Edwards MB, Dore CJ, Taylor KM. Tricuspid valve replacement: UK heart valve registry mid-term results comparing mechanical and biological prostheses. The Annals of Thoracic Surgery. 1998;**66**(6):1940-1947. DOI: 10.1016/s0003-4975(98)01183-7

[19] Rizzoli G, De Perini L, Bottio T, Minutolo G, Thiene G, Casarotto D. Prosthetic replacement of the tricuspid valve: Biological or mechanical? The Annals of Thoracic Surgery. 1998;**66**(6 Suppl):S62-S67. DOI: 10.1016/s0003-4975(98)01036-4

[20] Péterffy A, Szentkirályi I. Mechanical valves in tricuspid position: Cause of thrombosis and prevention. European Journal of Cardio-Thoracic Surgery. 2001;**19**(5):735-736. DOI: 10.1016/s1010-7940(01)00667-4

[21] Kaplan M, Kut MS, Demirtas MM, Cimen S, Ozler A. Prosthetic replacement of tricuspid valve: Bioprosthetic or mechanical. The Annals of Thoracic Surgery. 2002;**73**(2):467-473. DOI: 10.1016/s0003-4975(01)03128-9

[22] Joint Task Force on the Management of Valvular Heart Disease of the European Society of Cardiology (ESC), European Association for Cardio-Thoracic Surgery (EACTS), Vahanian A, Alfieri O, Andreotti F, Antunes MJ, et al. Guidelines on the management of valvular heart disease (version 2012). European Heart Journal. 2012;**33**(19):2451-2496. DOI: 10.1093/eurheartj/ehs109 Epub 2012 Aug 24

[23] Prihadi EA, Delgado V, Hahn RT, Leipsic J, Min JK, Bax JJ. Imaging needs

in novel Transcatheter tricuspid valve interventions. JACC: Cardiovascular Imaging. 2018;**11**(5):736-754. DOI: 10.1016/j.jcmg.2017.10.029

[24] Hahn RT. State-of-the-art review of echocardiographic imaging in the evaluation and treatment of functional tricuspid regurgitation. Circulation. Cardiovascular Imaging. 2016;**9**(12):e005332. DOI: 10.1161/CIRCIMAGING.116.005332

[25] Acar C, Ali M. Homologous transplantation of the mitral valve: A review. The Journal of Cardiovascular Surgery. 2004;**45**(5):455-464

[26] Hvass U, Baron F, Fourchy D, Pansard Y. Mitral homografts for total tricuspid valve replacement: Comparison of two techniques. The Journal of Thoracic and Cardiovascular Surgery. 2001;**121**(3):592-594. DOI: 10.1067/mtc.2001.110678

[27] Couetil JP, Argyriadis PG, Shafy A, Cohen A, Berrebi AJ, Loulmet DF, et al. Partial replacement of the tricuspid valve by mitral homografts in acute endocarditis. The Annals of Thoracic Surgery. 2002;**73**(6):1808-1812. DOI: 10.1016/s0003-4975(02)03574-9

[28] Kalangos A, Sierra J, Beghetti M, Trigo-Trindade P, Vala D, Christenson J. Tricuspid valve replacement with a mitral homograft in children with rheumatic tricuspid valvulopathy. The Journal of Thoracic and Cardiovascular Surgery. 2004;**127**(6):1682-1687. DOI: 10.1016/j.jtcvs.2003.12.030

[29] di Summa M, Donegani E, Zattera GF, Pansini S, Morea M. Successful orthotopic transplantation of a fresh tricuspid valve homograft in a human. The Annals of Thoracic Surgery. 1993;**56**(6):1407-1408. DOI: 10.1016/0003-4975(93)90698-h

[30] Campelos P, Encalada JF, Ramírez J, Pomar JL, Mestres CA. An old mitral homograft in the tricuspid position. The Journal of Heart Valve Disease. 2013;**22**(5):732-734

[31] Miyagishima RT, Brumwell ML, Eric Jamieson WR, Munt BI. Tricuspid valve replacement using a cryopreserved mitral homograft. Surgical technique and initial results. The Journal of Heart Valve Disease. 2000;**9**(6):805-808 discussion 808-9

[32] Ostrovsky Y, Spirydonau S, Shchatsinka M, Shket A. Surgical treatment of infective endocarditis with aortic and tricuspid valve involvement using cryopreserved aortic and mitral valve allografts. Interactive Cardiovascular and Thoracic Surgery. 2015;**20**(5):682-684. DOI: 10.1093/icvts/ivv028 Epub 2015 Feb 19

[33] Luciani GB, de Manna ND, Segreto A, Lanzoni L, Faggian G. Scalloped freehand pulmonary homograft for prosthetic tricuspid valve replacement. The Annals of Thoracic Surgery. 2021;**112**(1):e61-e64. DOI: 10.1016/j.athoracsur.2020.12.089 Epub 2021 Mar 1

[34] Dreyfus J, Audureau E, Bohbot Y, Coisne A, Lavie-Badie Y, Bouchery M, et al. TRI-SCORE: A new risk score for in-hospital mortality prediction after isolated tricuspid valve surgery. European Heart Journal. 2022;**43**(7):654-662. DOI: 10.1093/eurheartj/ehab679

[35] Nashef SA, Roques F, Sharples LD, Nilsson J, Smith C, Goldstone AR, et al. EuroSCORE II. European Journal of Cardio-Thoracic Surgery. 2012;**41**(4):734-744; discussion 744-5. DOI: 10.1093/ejcts/ezs043 Epub 2012 Feb 29

[36] Xu H, Wang H, Chen S, Chen Q, Xu T, Xu Z, et al. Prognostic value of modified model for end-stage liver

disease score in patients undergoing isolated tricuspid valve replacement. Front Cardiovasc Med. 2022;**9**:932142. DOI: 10.3389/fcvm.2022.932142

[37] Nuzhdin MD, Komarov RN, Matsuganov DA, Nadtochiy NB. Original technique for tricuspid valve replacement by mitral homograft: Step-by-step approach and initial results. Journal of Cardiac Surgery. 2022;**37**(12):5195-5201. DOI: 10.1111/jocs.17228 Epub 2022 Nov 15

[38] Mitchell C, Rahko PS, Blauwet LA, Canaday B, Finstuen JA, Foster MC, et al. Guidelines for performing a comprehensive transthoracic echocardiographic examination in adults: Recommendations from the American Society of Echocardiography. Journal of the American Society of Echocardiography. 2019;**32**(1):1-64. DOI: 10.1016/j.echo.2018.06.004 Epub 2018 Oct 1

[39] Akins CW, Miller DC, Turina MI, Kouchoukos NT, Blackstone EH, Grunkemeier GL, et al. Guidelines for reporting mortality and morbidity after cardiac valve interventions. European Journal of Cardio-Thoracic Surgery. 2008;**33**(4):523-528. DOI: 10.1016/j.ejcts.2007.12.055 Epub 2008 Mar 4

[40] Otto CM, Nishimura RA, Bonow RO, Carabello BA, Erwin JP 3rd, Gentile F, et al. 2020 ACC/AHA guideline for the Management of Patients with Valvular Heart Disease: A report of the American College of Cardiology/American Heart Association joint committee on clinical practice guidelines. Circulation. 2021;**143**(5):e72-e227. DOI: 10.1161/CIR.0000000000000923 Epub 2020 Dec 17. Erratum in: Circulation. 2021 Feb 2;**143**(5):e229

[41] Leviner DB, Friedman T, Zafrir B, Arazi M, Weis A, Bolotin G, et al. Midterm results of isolated tricuspid valve replacement-implications for clinical decision making. The Annals of Thoracic Surgery. 2022;**113**(3):793-799. DOI: 10.1016/j.athoracsur.2021.03.104 Epub 2021 Apr 25

[42] Mestres CA, Castellá M, Moreno A, Paré JC, del Rio A, Azqueta M, et al. Cryopreserved mitral homograft in the tricuspid position for infective endocarditis: A valve that can be repaired in the long-term (13 years). The Journal of Heart Valve Disease. 2006;**15**(3):389-391

[43] Pighi M, Pilati M, Pesarini G, Mammone C, Gottin L, Luciani GB, et al. Transcatheter valve-in-mitral homograft in tricuspid position: First-in-human report. The Canadian Journal of Cardiology. 2020;**36**(10):1690.e9-1690.e11. DOI: 10.1016/j.cjca.2020.04.027 Epub 2020 Apr 29

[44] Tudorache I, Horke A, Cebotari S, Sarikouch S, Boethig D, Breymann T, et al. Decellularized aortic homografts for aortic valve and aorta ascendens replacement. European Journal of Cardio-Thoracic Surgery. 2016;**50**(1):89-97. DOI: 10.1093/ejcts/ezw013 Epub 2016 Feb 18

[45] David TE, David C, Woo A, Manlhiot C. The Ross procedure: Outcomes at 20 years. The Journal of Thoracic and Cardiovascular Surgery. 2014;**147**(1):85-93. DOI: 10.1016/j.jtcvs.2013.08.007 Epub 2013 Sep 29

[46] Poynter JA, Eghtesady P, BW MC, Walters HL 3rd, Kirshbom PM, Blackstone EH, et al. Association of pulmonary conduit type and size with durability in infants and young children. The Annals of Thoracic Surgery. 2013;**96**(5):1695-1701; discussion 1701-2. DOI: 10.1016/j.athoracsur.2013.05.074 Epub 2013 Aug 22

[47] Batlivala SP, Emani S, Mayer JE, McElhinney DB. Pulmonary valve replacement function in adolescents: A comparison of bioprosthetic valves and homograft conduits. The Annals of Thoracic Surgery. 2012;**93**(6):2007-2016. DOI: 10.1016/j.athoracsur.2012.02.039 Epub 2012 May 4

[48] McNally RT, Brockbank KG. Issues surrounding the preservation of viable allograft heart valves. Journal of Medical Engineering & Technology. 1992;**16**(1):34-38. DOI: 10.3109/03091909209021955

[49] Elkins RC, Dawson PE, Goldstein S, Walsh SP, Black KS. Decellularized human valve allografts. The Annals of Thoracic Surgery. 2001;**71**(5 Suppl):S428-S432. DOI: 10.1016/s0003-4975(01)02503-6

Chapter 5

Clinical Implication of Cardiac Valve Allografts in Rare Surgical Circumstances

Roman Komarov, Mikhail D. Nuzhdin, Alisher Ismailbaev and Nikita Bashmakov

Abstract

The unique clinical and surgical experience with cardiac valve allografts is presented in the study. Cutting-edge approach with regard to clinical course of the disease, particular diagnostic findings, patient's preference, and allograft accessibility is highlighted in case series. State-of-the-art techniques, initial and mid-term results are summarized with a specific focus on allograft tissue application in cardiovascular surgery. Four patients underwent surgery during the period between February 2020 and February 2023 with inferior vena cava tumor involvement, destructive double valve endocarditis, rheumatic aortic and mitral insufficiency, and severe tricuspid regurgitation in patients with large ostium secundum and atrial fibrillation. All patients demonstrated an uneventful postoperative course.

Keywords: allograft, inferior vena cava, endocarditis, rheumatic heart disease, tricuspid replacement

1. Introduction

Cardiac valve allografts have been utilized since the late 1960s predominantly for surgical treatment of single valve infective endocarditis, rheumatic heart disease, and congenital valve anomalies [1–4]. The absence of strict indication, challenging surgical technique, along with allograft shortage used to prevent them from being widely acceptable in everyday clinical practice. Due to recent scientific advances in cardiac valve anatomy and physiology, development in surgical and preservation techniques, cardiac valve allografts have demonstrated their feasibility in those clinical scenarios where common valve substitutes have not shown significant clinical superiority [5]. Moreover, in some rare clinical circumstances, the choice between different valve prostheses might be a rather tough decision-making process regarding immediate and long-term results. In our study, we tried to summarize our experience with cardiac valve allografts in unusual clinical situations. The pulmonary artery trunk allograft in the surgical treatment of inferior vena cava tumor involvement, monoblock aorta-mitral homograft for destructive double valve endocarditis, mitral valve allograft in Bekhterev's disease, and mitral allograft (MA) for tricuspid replacement in a patient with large ostium secundum are consequently presented in our study. All four patients successfully underwent surgical repair in two departments with an uneventful postoperative course.

2. Case series description

2.1 Patient's population

During the period between February 2020 and February 2023, four patients underwent surgery due to different cardiac pathology at the two institutions ("Sechenov University" and "Chelyabinsk Regional Clinical Hospital"). All patients, their clinical course, and surgical interventions were considered exclusive regarding technique and cardiac valve allografts implanted. This study was approved by the Regional Ethics Committee of each hospital, and all patients signed their informed consent. The overall patient characteristic is depicted in **Table 1**.

2.2 Inferior vena cava replacement with pulmonary homograft

A 60-year-old woman with a clinical picture of dyspnea, weakness, and discomfort on moderate physical exertion was admitted to the Clinic of Faculty Surgery No. 1 of "Sechenov University". From the previous medical history, there was evidence of a left-sided hemicolectomy performed in 2017 for splenic flexure transverse colon cancer pT4AN2AM0 (TNM 8, histologically moderately differentiated adenocarcinoma). The patient was further operated on twice for liver metastases in 2018 (liver segments 2, 3, and 4A were resected) and in 2019 (liver segmentectomy IV b (the number of segment) was performed). The patient received a total of 8 courses of poly-chemotherapy. Initial investigation showed subtotal thrombosis of the right atrium due to tumor involvement of the vena cava and atrium wall. Contrast-enhanced computed tomography (CT) revealed a hepatic segment I metastasis with inferior vena cava thrombosis, spreading into the right atrial cavity. Thrombotic masses in the right atrial lumen were confirmed by transesophageal echocardiography (TEE).

The patient was scheduled for median sternotomy and upper median laparotomy approach that was performed on February 5, 2020. The stage of mobilization and removal of the first segment of the liver was performed before cardiopulmonary bypass. Standard ascending aorta, superior vena cava, and inferior vena cava in the infrahepatic segment bypass were initiated. After adhesiolysis, the superior vena cava and inferior vena cava (IVC) were snared, and a longitudinal cavatomy was performed. Invasion of the inferior vena cava wall into the tumorous process was revealed. Thrombotic masses were visualized that spread into the right atrium and were fixed to its wall; the tricuspid valve was intact. Radical excision of the tumor masses entailed resectioning the right atrium and inferior vena cava area with subsequent replacement of the part of inferior vena cava and right atrium wall with a cryopreserved pulmonary homograft (28 mm in diameter). The cardiopulmonary bypass time was 67 minutes. The resected tumor, inferior vena cava, and the final view after reconstruction are shown in **Figures 1** and **2**.

In the 3-year follow-up period, transthoracic echocardiography and contrast-enhanced CT depicted no evidence of tumor recurrence.

	Age (year)/sex	Primary pathology	Homograft type utilized	Cardiac structure replaced	30-Day mortality	Complication	Follow-up period, month	Mid-term survival
Patient 1	60/F	Metastatic liver cancer	Pulmonary trunk	Inferior vena cava and right atrium	—	—	36	Survived
Patient 2	56/M	Double valve infective endocarditis	Aortomitral block	Aortic root and mitral valve	—	—	6	Survived
Patient 3	52/F	Bekhterev's disease	Mitral valve	Mitral valve	—	—	12	Survived
Patient 4	44/F	Large secondary ASD and severe tricuspid regurgitation	Mitral homograft	Tricuspid valve	—	—	4	Survived

Table 1.
The overall patient's characteristic.

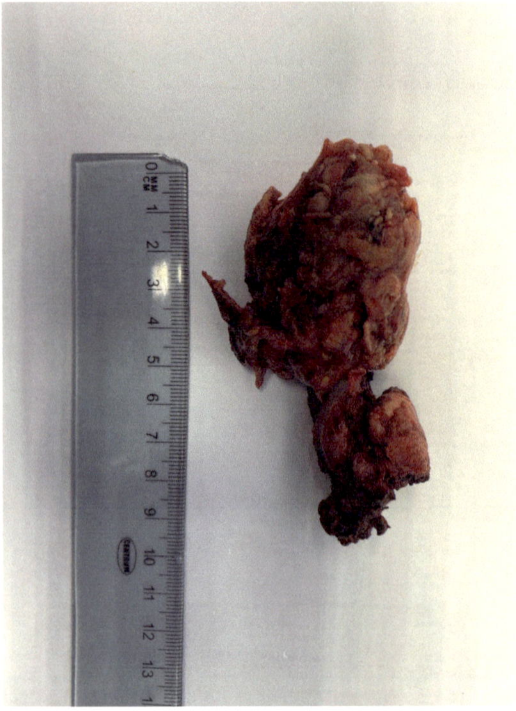

Figure 1.
Intraoperative view. Tumor mass deleted from the inferior vena cava.

2.3 Double valve destructive infective endocarditis treatment with monoblock aortomitral homograft implantation

A 56-year-old male patient with subacute infective endocarditis (presumably from September 2021) with aortic (severe failure) and mitral (severe failure) valve involvement and aortic root abscess was operated on in June 2022. The patient had a commonplace clinical course of infective endocarditis that had been confirmed under current guidelines before admission. Considering the limited but promising world experience with monobloc aorta-mitral homografts, we assumed that monobloc aortomitral homograft implantation could be an alternative to the "standard" Commando procedure. The median sternotomy approach and standard cardiopulmonary bypass with bicaval cannulation and cold cardioplegia. This technique used in our clinic entailed several steps described below.

2.3.1 Technique of aortomitral homograft implantation

1. After the transverse aortotomy, the inspection of aortic valve revealed total leaflet destruction, vegetation, and abscess cavity on the level of aortic annulus. The valve was excised, and total root debridement was performed in order to get rid of infected and necrotic masses. Then deep mobilization of the aortic root, excision of valsalva sinus, and coronary arteries mobilization. From the middle of the noncoronary sinus, an incision was made down to the anterior mitral valve leaflet. The left atrial roof was opened. For better exposure of the mitral

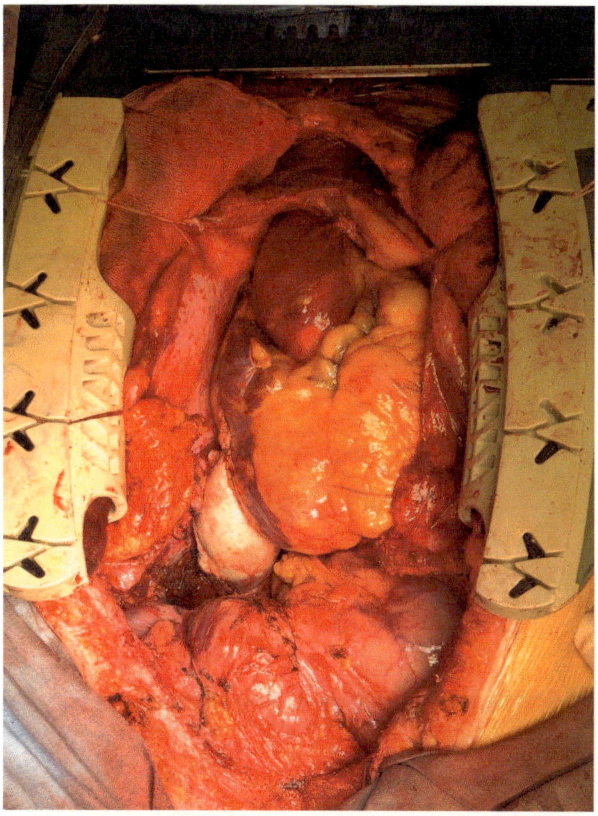

Figure 2.
The final view. Inferior vena cava replaced by pulmonary allograft.

valve, the incision of the left atrium can be extended by dissecting the interatrial septum and the right atrium (**Figure 3**).

2. Having the mitral valve excised, the aortomitral homograft was fixed in the mitral position. The homograft was sewn first along the posterior annulus, then along the anterior one. In the area of the aortomitral junction, homograft sutures were placed oriented to the fibrous triangles, and one suture was placed to capture the aortic fibrous ring tissue, in order to close it (**Figure 4**).

3. The papillary muscles of the homograft were anastomosed side-by-side to corresponding papillary muscles with four interrupted stitches using "Ethibond" 3-0 sutures. The aortic part of the homograft was inserted into the left ventricle (LV cavity and was sewn into the aortic root position afterward (**Figure 5**).

4. The aortic homograft is everted from the LV; the coronary artery mouths are implanted into the homograft. Posterior partial ring mitral homograft annuloplasty is performed (**Figure 6**).

Cardiopulmonary bypass time was 235 minutes; myocardial ischemia time was 210 minutes. The patient was in the intensive care unit for 3 days and in the hospital

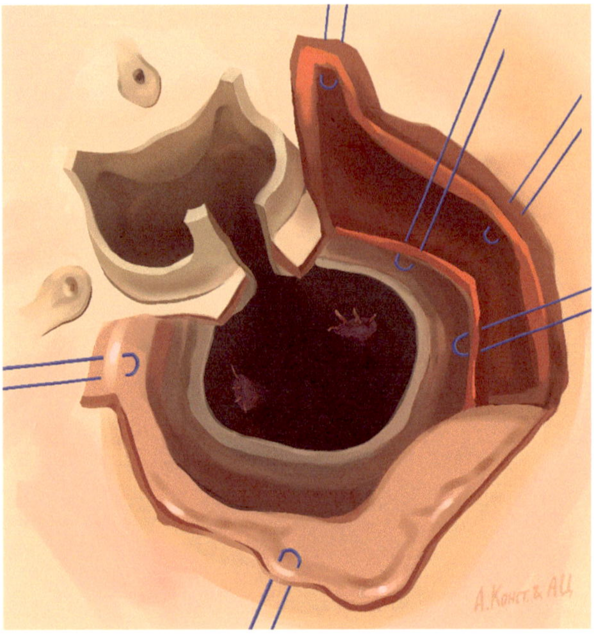

Figure 3.
Aortic and mitral valve are excised. The incision of the left atrium is extended by dissecting the interatrial septum and the right atrium.

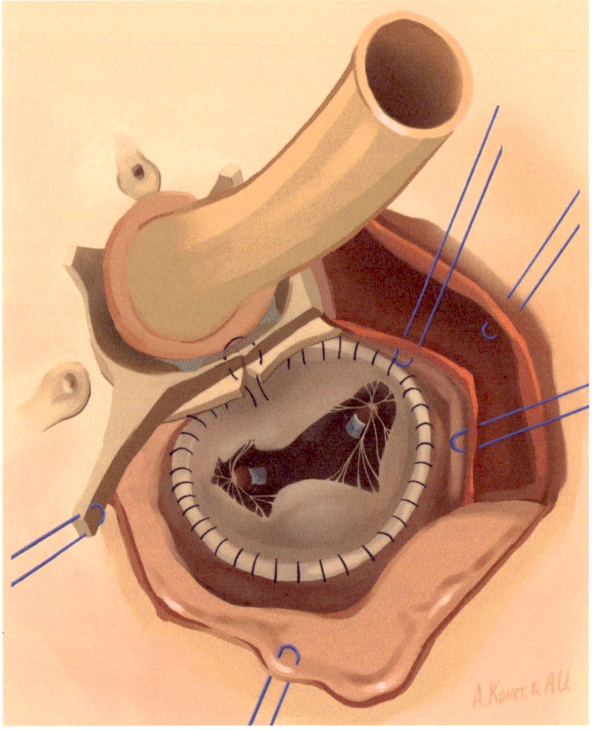

Figure 4.
The aortomitral homograft is fixed in the mitral position.

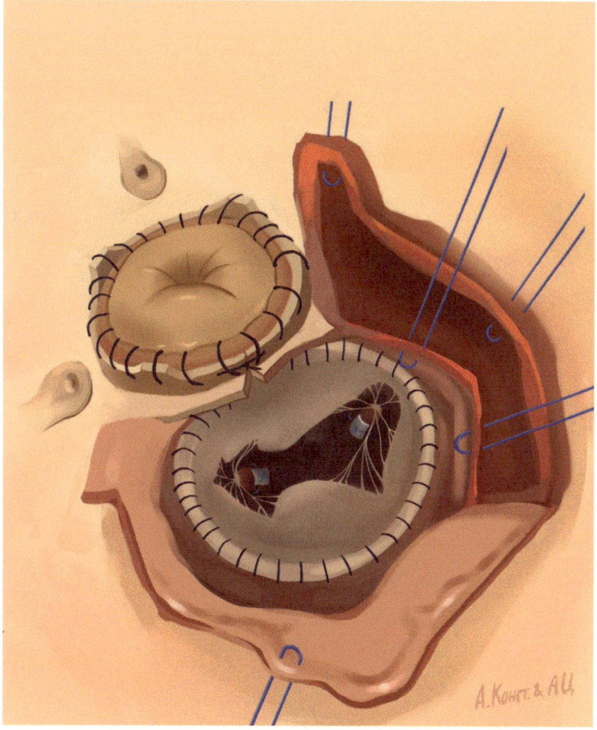

Figure 5.
The aortic part of the homograft is inserted into the left ventricle (LV cavity) and is sewn into the aortic root position.

for 12 days. In the postoperative period, the patient underwent echocardiography assessment and was discharged from the hospital with excellent homograft function.

2.4 Concomitant homograft mitral valve replacement and aortic autopericardial neo-cuspidalization in patient with Bekhterev's disease

A 52-year-old woman with Bekhterev's disease was admitted to the Department of Cardiac Surgery ("Sechenov University") for elective aortic and mitral valve surgery. On admission, the patient's clinical status was presented with pronounced dyspnea at rest, cough, increased fatigue, and moderate pain in the heart area. From the past medical history, we found out that the first manifestation of Bekhterev's disease occurred at the age of 25 with iridocyclitis, which at that time was regarded as a manifestation of herpes-virus infection. At age 42, the presence of the HLA B-27 gene was laboratory confirmed. Back in those days, mild-to-moderate mitral regurgitation was revealed. Four years later, at the age of 46, transthoracic echocardiography showed mild aortic regurgitation. Sulfasalazine was first prescribed in a dosage of 1 g two times a day. In 2022, at the age of 52, after a coronavirus infection, patient's condition went to decline with increased dyspnea and swelling of the lower extremities. Heart auscultation revealed a diastolic murmur, mainly in the area of the aorta, and a systolic noise irradiating to the left axillary region. Spinal mobility was limited due to stiffness in the lower back and in the cervical region. Transthoracic echocardiogram showed enlarged LV (LV end-diastolic diameter 57 mm, end-diastolic volume 190 ml), LV EF at rest 58%,

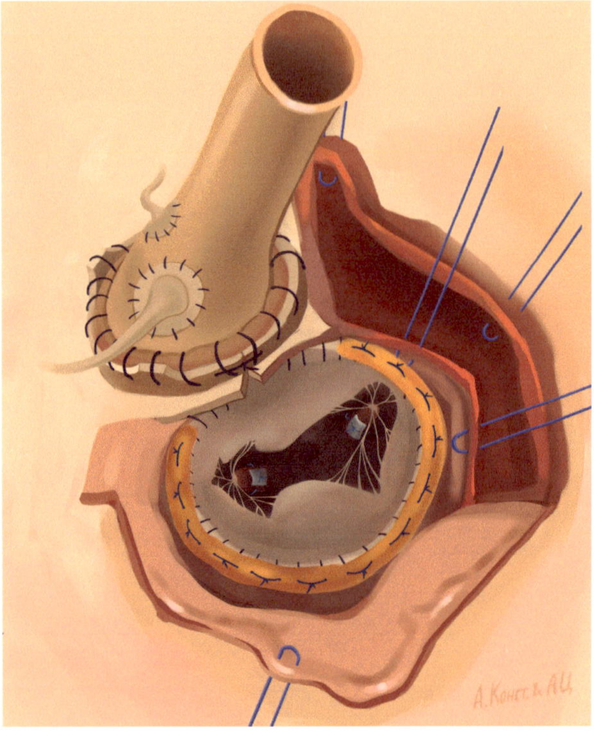

Figure 6.
Posterior partial ring mitral homograft annuloplasty is performed. Final view.

thickened aortic root wall, marginal fibrosis of aortic valve cusps, right coronary cusp thickened, central coaptation defect, and restricted leaflet motion. The mitral valve leaflets were thickened with restricted motion as well. The doppler-echocardiography confirmed severe central aortic regurgitation and severe mitral insufficiency.

2.4.1 Surgical homograft mitral valve replacement and aortic autopericardial neo-cuspidalization

Instead of the mechanical double valve replacement, the autopericardial neocuspidization was opted for aortic valve procedure, while MA was chosen for mitral valve replacement. After the median sternotomy a pericardial flap was harvested with its subsequent preservation in 0.6% glutaraldehyde. Standard cardiopulmonary bypass and cold cardioplegia were applied. Intraoperative assessment revealed bicuspid aortic valve pathology with leaflet fibrosis. Mitral valve leaflets were also significantly thickened and were not considered for mitral repair. Three semilunar cusps of the same size were dissected from the pericardial flap. The aortic valve neocuspidization with autologous pericardium leaflets was performed. The autopericardium valve was formed (**Figure 7a**). The next step was mitral homograft implantation in the mitral position (**Figure 7b**). The mitral homograft papillary muscles were fixed to the LV papillary muscles with four U-shaped sutures using 4-0 sutures. The mitral homograft was placed into the LV cavity, then mitral homograft was fixed to the mitral annulus with continuous 5-0 polypropylene sutures (**Figure 7c**). The posterior mitral annulus was reinforced with soft band (**Figure 7d**). TEE and postoperative

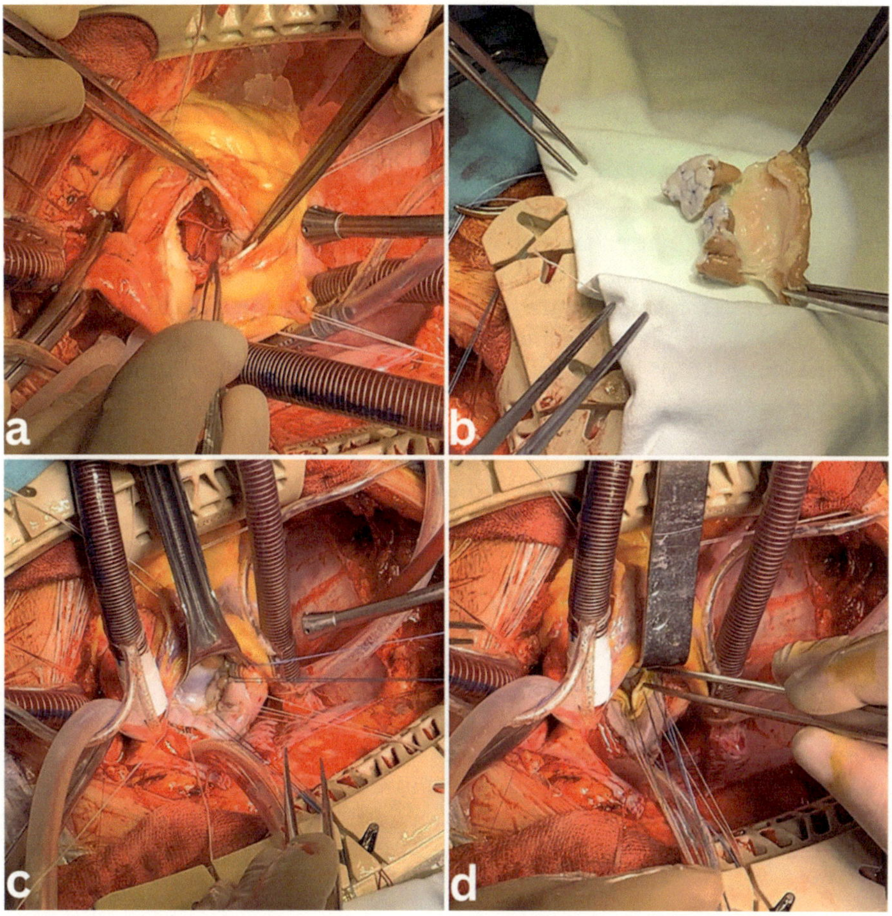

Figure 7.
(a) Aortic valve replacement with autopericardial neo-cuspidalization; (b) mitral allograft; (c) mitral allograft in mitral position; (d) ring implantation.

echocardiography showed improved function of aortic autopericardial neovalve and mitral homograft with only trivial regurgitation. The duration of cardio-pulmonary bypass (CPB) was 182 min, and the aortic cross-clamp duration was 155 min. The patient was discharged on the 14th day after surgery in satisfactory condition, with marked increase in physical tolerance and decreased dyspnea. Transthoracic echocardiography 1 year after the operation shows mild MA regurgitation with peak pressure gradient of 3 mmHg, mean pressure gradient of 2 mmHg, and trivial aortic regurgitation with peak pressure gradient of 8 mmHg, mean pressure gradient of 4 mmHg.

2.5 Homograft tricuspid valve replacement with large atrium septum defect closure and cryoablation procedure in adult

A 40-year-old woman was admitted to the Chelyabinsk Regional Clinical Hospital with severe tricuspid regurgitation, large atrial septal defect (ASD), signs of right sided-heart failure, and persistent atrial fibrillation. The patient reported progressive exercise-induced shortness of breath (New York Heart Association functional class III) during the last 6 months after she had documented the first episode of AF.

2.5.1 Diagnostic assessment

Initial diagnostic workup by echocardiography confirmed large ASD (46 mm), severely dilated right atrium—65 × 81 mm, and right ventricle (RV) – 52 mm, PH of 60 mmHg and severe tricuspid regurgitation (vena contracta—9 mm, regurgitant volume—83 ml). A contrast-enhanced cardiac computed tomography (CCT) revealed a large ostium secundum (53 × 43 mm, 17 cm^2) (**Figure 8**), severely dilated RV (end-diastolic volume of 550 ml, end-systolic volume of 355 ml), and reduced ejection fraction (EF) of 35%, right ventricle fractional area contraction (RV FAC)—25%, tricuspid annulus plane systolic excursion (TAPSE)—10 mm. The patient was scheduled for concomitant surgery. Having discussed all available options for tricuspid surgery, patient's informed concern was obtained with regard to either annuloplasty or homograft replacement. The patient refused either mechanical or stented biological prosthesis because of personal and religious beliefs.

2.5.2 Surgical procedure

Concomitant operation was performed through the medial sternotomy approach with standard cardiopulmonary bypass. The cryoablation procedure was carried before valve repair. TV inspection revealed severely dilated annulus, leaflet shrinkage, and thickening that was assumed to be not appropriate for successful repair. MA was chosen as a valve substitute. ASD was closed by means of a bovine pericardium patch of appropriate size. After several measures had been taken, MA was implanted in the tricuspid orifice. The procedure was accompanied by tricuspid ring implantation. Intraoperative echocardiography (ECHO) demonstrated no residual regurgitation on MA with mean diastolic pressure gradient of 2 mmHg.

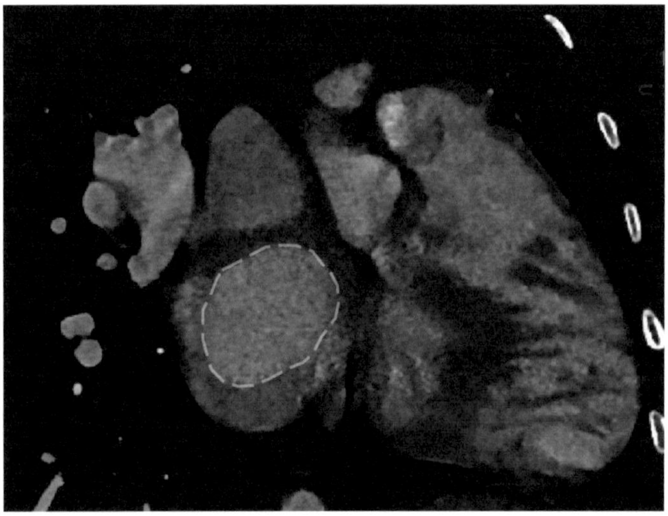

Figure 8.
ECG-gated cardiac CT reformation in interventricular septum plane before operation, mid diastole. Large ASD in the central part of interatrial septum.

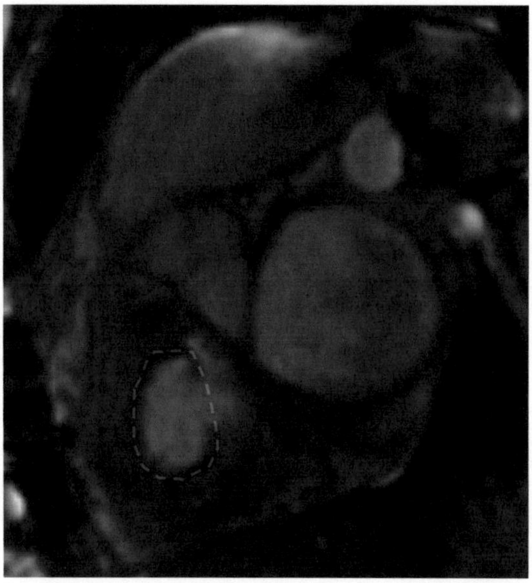

Figure 9.
Short-axis steady-state free precession cardiac MRI in tricuspid plane, diastole. Homograft annulus after surgery. The dashed line indicates valve annulus with annuloplasty ring.

2.5.3 Postoperative follow-up

Postoperative CCT demonstrated reduction in RV volumes with EF of 47%, RV FAC—34% and TAPSE—16 mm. Homograft orifice area was 9 cm^2 and excellent leaflet coaptation was clearly seen (**Figure 9**). TTE demonstrated mean trans-homograft pressure gradient 1.4 mmHg, normal leaflet motion without regurgitation (**Figure 10**). Patient was discharged from the hospital with sinus rhythm and excellent homograft function. Oral anticoagulation therapy was stopped after a 3-month period of intake.

3. Discussion

Cardiac valve allografts have been thought to be plausible valve substitutes in wide spectrum of surgical scenarios. In addition, it is also believed that allograft's availability enables to broad technical opportunities [5, 6]. Regarding radical treatment of hepatocellular carcinoma with tumor thrombi in the inferior vena cava or right atrium, surgical removal of thrombotic masses from the inferior vena cava and the right atrium remains to the most efficient method of treatment that can reduce the risk of systemic metastasis and sudden death due to pulmonary thromboembolism or occlusion of the tricuspid valve by a tumor thrombus [7]. Without surgical repair, the median survival is less than 12 months, and chemotherapy has not demonstrated acceptable survival [8, 9]. Descriptive and comparative analysis of different types of allograft tissue in inferior vena cava replacement has not been provided in available databases. Arterial and venous allografts could also be considered feasible prosthetic material, although pulmonary homograft conduit was optimal for two main reasons. Firstly, pulmonary allograft was available for subsequent use. Secondly, a bigger size

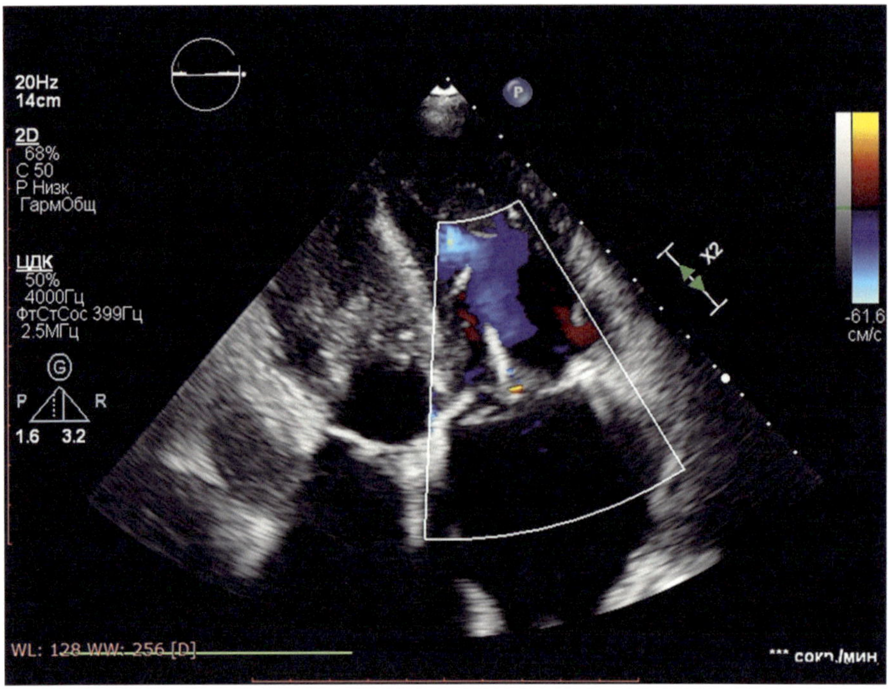

Figure 10.
Postoperative TTE. Apical 4-chamber view. Excellent leaflet coaptation without residual regurgitation on mitral homograft in tricuspid position.

of pulmonary conduit seemed to be more advantageous for dilated patient's inferior vena cava and more suitable for right atrium reconstruction. Nevertheless, diverse spectrum of allograft tissue conduits should be carefully investigated in such procedures. Our experience suggests in favor of radical surgical treatment where allograft tissue demonstrated its relevant implication with excellent results.

Another challenging circumstance is destructive double valve infective endocarditis with central fibrous body involvement. There are no systematic results of aortomitral homograft implantation for such patients, and these operations are rarely performed [10, 11]. Theoretically, the main advantages of the method are the absence of synthetic material and no need for anticoagulation. Another potential benefit of the aortomitral homograft is the preservation of mobility of the supporting apparatus, which may be important for long-term homograft function and cardiac performance. Mechanical valves remain the most commonly used substitute for double valve replacement, still carrying the high risk of bleeding and thromboembolic events in the long run. Potential benefits of allografts in favor of re-infection resistance have not been proved in randomized trials; by the way, such trials are limited. Current clinical guidelines are inconclusive regarding valve choice in different clinical scenarios, which formally enables the heart team to create their own strategy based on the patient's clinical status, urgency, and graft availability. From our point of expertise, allograft double valve replacement might well be taken into account, given full respect to obvious benefits and potential drawbacks in the mid- and long-term.

Concomitant cardiac procedures with cardiac valve allografts are rare and have not been described precisely. Cardiac involvement in Bekhterev's disease usually manifests as aortic insufficiency, aortitis, or cardiac conduction abnormalities. Mitral insufficiency is less commonly defined, predominantly when subaortic fibrosis reaches the anterior mitral valve leaflet [12, 13]. Experience with mitral homograft implantation has shown that valve lesions of rheumatic etiology, which include Bekhterev's disease, may be a major indication for this technique [14]. When it comes to the method of aortic valve repair, there was a choice between a biological valve, the Ross procedure, and neocuspidization, because the patient avoided anticoagulation. Low durability of the Ross procedure in rheumatic disorders may be due to autoimmune response to type IV collagen, which is contained in the valve leaflets [15]. The experience with biological valves in rheumatic diseases is similarly unsatisfactory, with early degeneration and an increased risk of reoperation [16]. We reckon that allografts and reconstructive surgery using autologous materials provide a better hemodynamic profile along with avoidance of lifelong anticoagulation therapy. Autopericardial neocuspidization could be under the scope of surgical interest, regarding their potential "bridging" role in reconstructive surgery, avoiding anticoagulation-related complications and enabling more radical surgery (allograft root replacement) or transcatheter aortic valve replacement in long-term.

Considering MAs application in reconstructive tricuspid surgery, there is a sustained interest in terms of superior initial results, high hemodynamic performance, and potentially lower risk of complication in long-term follow-up [1, 17, 18]. A recent meta-analysis shows neither biological nor mechanical prosthesis provide satisfactory early and long-term results [19, 20]. MA could probably outweigh biological prosthesis in hemodynamic performance and long-term outcomes, but the data is confined to few clinical studies but with promising initial results, which encourage wider acceptance of MA in tricuspid position. Moreover, in cases where tricuspid repair cannot be performed, current guidelines and markets give no particular feedback regarding prosthetic choice, and stented biological valves along with mechanical are still recommended. Our study gives practical insight into feasibility of MA in the treatment of degenerative TV pathology in patients who does not accept traditional prosthetic options. Concomitant cryoablation for atrial fibrillation in combination with homograft implantation has not been described in available databases.

4. Conclusion

Assuming our surgical experience with cardiac valve allografts in unusual clinical cases, we can conclude that allograft valves might take place as a plausible prosthetic tissue in a wide spectrum of diseases. Marked hemodynamic performance and excellent early and mid-term results could be achieved with low risk of complications and zero mortality in selected patients. Technical procedure-related challenges could be confidently resolved by having pliable allograft material available at the time of operation. Patient's desires and preferences still play a crucial role in decision-making. Further investigations are needed to prove potential benefits of allografts in cardiovascular surgery.

Conflict of interest

The authors declare no conflict of interest.

Author details

Roman Komarov[1]*, Mikhail D. Nuzhdin[2], Alisher Ismailbaev[1] and Nikita Bashmakov[1]

1 Clinic for Aortic and Cardio-Vascular Surgery, Federal State Autonomous Educational Institution of Higher Education First Moscow State Medical University Named after I.M. Sechenova of the Ministry of Health of the Russian Federation (Sechenov University), Moscow, Russian Federation

2 State Budgetary Healthcare Institution "Chelyabinsk Regional Clinical Hospital", Chelyabinsk, Russian Federation

*Address all correspondence to: drkomarov1977@gmail.com

References

[1] Nappi F, Spadaccio C, Acar C. Use of allogeneic tissue to treat infective valvular disease: has everything been said? The Journal of Thoracic and Cardiovascular Surgery 2017;**153**(4): 824-828. DOI: 10.1016/j.jtcvs.2016.09.071. Epub 2016 Oct 24. PMID: 27866779

[2] Kirklin JK. Challenging homografts as the holy grail for aortic valve endocarditis. The Journal of Thoracic and Cardiovascular Surgery 2016;**151**(5):1230-1231. DOI: 10.1016/j.jtcvs.2015.12.009. Epub 2015 Dec 13. PMID: 26778216

[3] Kim JB, Ejiofor JI, Yammine M, Camuso JM, Walsh CW, Ando M, Melnitchouk SI, Rawn JD, Leacche M, MacGillivray TE, Cohn LH, Byrne JG, Sundt TM. Are homografts superior to conventional prosthetic valves in the setting of infective endocarditis involving the aortic valve? The Journal of Thoracic and Cardiovascular Surgery 2016;**151**(5):1239-46, 1248.e1-2. DOI: 10.1016/j.jtcvs.2015.12.061. Epub 2016 Jan 23. PMID: 26936004

[4] Kalangos A, Sierra J, Beghetti M, Trigo-Trindade P, Vala D, Christenson J. Tricuspid valve replacement with a mitral homograft in children with rheumatic tricuspid valvulopathy. The Journal of Thoracic and Cardiovascular Surgery. 2004;**127**(6):1682-1687. DOI: 10.1016/j.jtcvs.2003.12.030 PMID: 15173724

[5] Yousif A, Ali K, Anssar M, Harringer W, El-Essawi A, Brouwer R. A 20-year experience with cryopreserved allografts as the valve replacement of choice in aortic root reconstruction for destructive endocarditis with abscess formation. Interactive Cardiovascular and Thoracic Surgery. 2022. DOI: 10.1093/icvts/ivac188

[6] Shrestha BM, Fukushima S, Vrtik M, Chong IH, Sparks L, Jalali H, et al. Partial replacement of tricuspid valve using cryopreserved homograft. The Annals of Thoracic Surgery. 2010;**89**(4):1187-1194. DOI: 10.1016/j.athoracsur.2009.12.047 PMID: 20338330

[7] Wakayama K, Kamiyama T, Yokoo H, Kakisaka T, Kamachi H, Tsuruga Y, et al. Surgical management of hepatocellular carcinoma with tumor thrombi in the inferior vena cava or right atrium. World Journal of Surgical Oncology. 2013;**11**:259. DOI: 10.1186/1477-7819-11-259. PMID: 24093164; PMCID: PMC3851861

[8] Rougier P, Milan C, Lazorthes F, Fourtanier G, Partensky C, Baumel H, et al. Prospective study of prognostic factors in patients with unresected hepatic metastases from colorectal cancer. Fondation Française de Cancérologie Digestive. The British Journal of Surgery. 1995;**82**(10):1397-1400. DOI: 10.1002/bjs.1800821034 PMID: 7489177

[9] Isenberg J, Fischbach R, Krüger I, Keller HW. Treatment of liver metastases from colorectal cancer. Anticancer Research. 1996;**16**(3A):1291-1295. PMID: 8702252

[10] Hosseini MT, Kourliouros A, Sarsam M. Double-valve endocarditis homograft and patch repair. The Annals of Thoracic Surgery. 2009;**88**(5):1708-1709. DOI: 10.1016/j.athoracsur.2009.02.041 PMID: 19853153

[11] Elgharably H, Hakim AH, Unai S, Hussain ST, Shrestha NK, Gordon S, et al. The incorporated aortomitral homograft for double-valve endocarditis: the 'hemi-Commando' procedure. Early

and mid-term outcomes. European Journal of Cardio-Thoracic Surgery. 2018;**53**(5):1055-1061. DOI: 10.1093/ejcts/ezx439 PMID: 29253091

[12] Atzeni F, Nucera V, Galloway J, Zoltán S, Nurmohamed M. Cardiovascular risk in ankylosing spondylitis and the effect of anti-TNF drugs: a narrative review. Expert Opinion on Biological Therapy 2020;**20**(5):517-524. DOI: 10.1080/14712598.2020.1704727. Epub 2019 Dec 17. PMID: 31847607

[13] Ward MM, Deodhar A, Akl EA, Lui A, Ermann J, Gensler LS, Smith JA, et al. American College of Rheumatology/Spondylitis Association of America/Spondyloarthritis Research and Treatment Network 2015 recommendations for the treatment of ankylosing spondylitis and nonradiographic axial spondyloarthritis. Arthritis Care & Research. 2016;**68**(2):151-166. DOI: 10.1002/acr.22708. Epub 2015 Sep 24. PMID: 26401907; PMCID: PMC5123844

[14] Acar C. The mitral homograft-is it worthwhile? The Journal of Thoracic and Cardiovascular Surgery. 2000;**120**(3):448-449. DOI: 10.1067/mtc.2000.109924 PMID: 10962403

[15] Tandon R, Sharma M, Chandrashekhar Y, Kotb M, Yacoub MH, Narula J. Revisiting the pathogenesis of rheumatic fever and carditis. Nature Reviews. Cardiology 2013;**10**(3):171-177. DOI: 10.1038/nrcardio.2012.197. Epub 2013 Jan 15. PMID: 23319102

[16] Yu J, Wang W, Bioprosthetic vs. Mechanical mitral valve replacement for rheumatic heart disease in patients aged 50-70 years. Frontiers in Cardiovascular Medicine. 2022;**9**:904958. DOI: 10.3389/fcvm.2022.904958 PMID: 35711344; PMCID: PMC9193579

[17] Nuzhdin MD, Komarov RN, Matsuganov DA, Nadtochiy NB. Original technique for tricuspid valve replacement by mitral homograft: step-by-step approach and initial results. Journal of Cardiac Surgery 2022;**37**(12):5195-5201. DOI: 10.1111/jocs.17228. Epub 2022 Nov 15. PMID: 36378863

[18] Olivito S, Lalande S, Nappi F, Hammoudi N, D'Alessandro C, Fouret P, Acar C. Structural deterioration of the cryopreserved mitral homograft valve. The Journal of Thoracic and Cardiovascular Surgery. 2012;**144**(2):313-320, 320.e1. DOI: 10.1016/j.jtcvs.2011.06.041. Epub 2011 Sep 8. PMID: 21855094

[19] Cheng Z, Fang T, Wang D, Guo Y. Tricuspid valve replacement: mechanical or biological prostheses? A systematic review and meta-analysis. The Heart Surgery Forum. 2021;**24**(2):E209-E214. DOI: 10.1532/hsf.3531

[20] Leviner DB, Friedman T, Zafrir B, Arazi M, Weis A, Bolotin G, Sharoni E. Midterm results of isolated tricuspid valve replacement-implications for clinical decision making. The Annals of Thoracic Surgery 2022;**113**(3):793-799. DOI: 10.1016/j.athoracsur.2021.03.104. Epub 2021 Apr 25. PMID: 33910052

Chapter 6

Defining Success and Ethical Decision-Making in Vascularized Composite Allotransplantation: A Bioethical Deliberation Model

Anneke Farías-Yapur

Abstract

This chapter explores the intricate bioethical considerations surrounding Vascularized Composite Allotransplantation (VCA) and proposes a bioethical deliberation model. The primary focus is on defining success criteria for VCA and fostering ethical decision-making to enhance patient outcomes. The chapter delves into critical variables to define beneficence, non-maleficence, autonomy, and justice and their role in shaping the success of VCA procedures. The significance of assessing both receiver and institutional capacities is emphasized, along with the importance of objective resilience, deferential vulnerability, and decisional capacity in evaluating patient eligibility. Furthermore, the healthcare team's capacity for ethical deliberation and the resources required to support patient resilience are explored. By addressing these crucial factors, the proposed bioethical deliberation model aims to align VCA practices with the principles of beneficence, non-maleficence, autonomy, and justice. This chapter offers valuable insights into the ethical dimensions of VCA and provides a framework that can contribute to improved patient care and treatment outcomes.

Keywords: ethical decision-making, Vascularized Composite Allotransplantation, success criteria, objective resilience, bioethical deliberation

1. Introduction

Vascularized Composite Allotransplantation (VCA) is a surgical technique aimed at transplanting multiple tissues as a single functional unit, such as skin, muscles, nerves, and bone, with the objective of enhancing the quality of life. Despite significant advancements in surgical techniques, several bioethical challenges remain to be addressed. These challenges encompass various aspects, including the economic burdens associated with the procedure [1], the potential risks of long-term immunosuppressive therapy, such as increased susceptibility to malignancy [2], and the occurrence of acute and chronic rejection [3, 4]. Moreover, the autonomy of patients in choosing a non-life-saving intervention [5] and the

IntechOpen

adequacy of psychosocial evaluation tools developed primarily in developed countries [6] are important considerations in the ethical discourse surrounding VCA. Additionally, bioethical concerns extend to the capacity of healthcare teams to effectively manage VCA cases and the need to balance patient suitability for the procedure with the capacity of the country and healthcare system to support such interventions. Finally, definitions regarding transplant success are not straightforward [7]. Although it is true that definitions of transplant success may vary depending on each individual, we believe there must be core domains upon which individual traits can be accommodated.

To address these important considerations, it is crucial to define the success criteria for VCA and establish a framework for evaluating patients, healthcare systems, and the bioethical aspects involved. This chapter aims to examine the bioethical considerations in VCA and propose a preliminary bioethical deliberation model. To achieve this, first, we will try to define success criteria for VCA procedures, based on critical variables that operationalize the principles of beneficence, non-maleficence, autonomy, and justice. Based on the definition of success, a bioethical deliberation model is proposed to evaluate Deliberative Capacity (to attend to the criteria of Autonomy and Justice), as well as Receiver-Offering Capacity (to attend to the criteria of Nonmaleficence and Beneficence), both on patients and healthcare teams. By addressing these bioethical considerations and providing a clear framework for decision-making, the aim is to ensure that VCA procedures are conducted in an ethically responsible manner, considering the well-being of patients and the integrity of healthcare systems.

2. Towards a definition of success in VCA

To approach a comprehensive definition of success in VCA, it is essential to consider the four fundamental principles of beneficence, nonmaleficence, autonomy, and justice, with critical variables serving as a solid foundation for defining and operationalizing these principles.

2.1 Non-maleficence and beneficence

To precisely define the concept of beneficence in the context of VCA, it is essential to revisit the procedure's bioethical justification: the enhancement of quality of life. Quality of life is intricately tied to the processes of multisystemic resilience, which enables individuals and their support networks to cope with adversity and continue pursuing their goals and aspirations despite challenges.

The focus on resilience as a key variable for success should guide bioethical deliberation. We propose to pay special focus on Objective Resilience, as an indicator that encompasses both key multisystemic resilience domains, as well as important quality of life domains as measured by the WHOQOL [8] and SF-36 [9]. Therefore, it is important to define what multisystemic and objective resilience entails.

2.1.1 Multisystemic resilience

According to Ungar [10], resilience is a complex and multisystemic phenomenon that extends beyond individual characteristics. It recognizes that an individual's ability to navigate and overcome adversity is intricately tied to the availability, accessibility, and meaningfulness of critical resources within various systems that encompass different domains of life that directly or indirectly impact an individual's ability to navigate and overcome adversity. According to Bronfenbrenner's Theory of Social Ecology [11], these systems include the individual, their close support networks such as family and healthcare teams (microsystem), the interactions between different microsystems (mesosystem), broader social structures that influence meso- and microsystemic relationships (exosystem), cultural norms, laws, and customs (macrosystem), and the temporal dimension within which these systems interact and change (cronosystem).

This multisystemic perspective allows individuals or communities to engage in processes of recovery, adaptation, and transformation. Recovery, as described by Ungar [10], involves returning to a state equal to or better than before the adversity. It signifies the ability to regain equilibrium and restore functioning after experiencing challenges. Adaptation, on the other hand, refers to the process of positively adjusting to changes brought about by adversity. It entails developing new strategies, skills, and perspectives to effectively cope and thrive in the face of challenges. Lastly, transformation occurs when systems are improved as a result of navigating and overcoming adversity. It signifies the potential for growth, innovation, and positive change within individuals, communities, and even larger societal structures.

2.1.2 QoL-objective resilience

Resilience, at any level, is achieved through the availability, accessibility, and meaningfulness of critical resources within multiple systems. This inherently multisystemic nature of resilience forms the foundation for objective resilience. Objective resilience, as emphasized in the bioethical deliberation model, encompasses both immediate contextual domains that directly support QoL—such as support network's material stability, access to environment, independence in relation to physical and emotional limitations, and social functioning—as well as individual domains, such as physical pain, physical energy, physical limitations, psychological well-being, psychological limitations, and individual material stability. These dimensions provide a comprehensive understanding of an individual's overall functioning and the impact of different factors on their quality of life.

By considering these factors, objective resilience serves as a critical material variable that underpins the moral justification of VCA. The underlying promise of VCA is to improve resilience via the increase of availability, accessibility, or meaningfulness of critical resources both for objective resilience domains, as well as those of multisystemic resilience. Thus, defining transplant success involves increasing objective and multisystemic resilience not only in terms of recovery, primarily through treatment adherence, but also in the patient's adaptation and the transformation of the healthcare system.

2.2 Autonomy

Autonomy, a fundamental principle of bioethics, plays a vital role in informed consent and medical practice. Autonomy is characterized by self-governance and personal causation, reflecting an individual's ability to make autonomous choices. Respecting patient autonomy plays a crucial role in defining the success of a transplant as it recognizes their ability to deliberate and make decisions regarding their treatment [12]. Autonomy forms the foundation for informed consent to be considered valid [13–15]. Several factors must be evaluated by practitioners to determine the validity of patients' informed consent, including competence, disclosure, comprehension, voluntariness, and agreement [13].

Psychological assessments are commonly used to assess the capacity of transplant candidates to provide informed consent. However, these assessments primarily focus on cognitive vulnerabilities that may impede understanding. While voluntariness and agreement are essential aspects of informed consent, the psychological factors involved are often overlooked due to their challenging measurability and susceptibility to deferential vulnerability: pressures that prompt patients to "accede to the perceived desires of certain others notwithstanding an inner reticence to do so" [16]. Such vulnerability—among others—compromise consent. Despite its relevance, currently, psychosocial evaluations of patient candidacy do not specifically address the assessment of autonomy in relation to deferential vulnerabilities [17]. To bridge this gap, we propose and continue developing a theoretical framework (*under review*) informed by a Kantian interpretation of Honneth's Recognition Theory [18, 19], emphasizing the importance of self-relationships and human dignity. This framework is complemented by **Figure 1**, which shows key moments of the theory, as well as indicators for its observation.

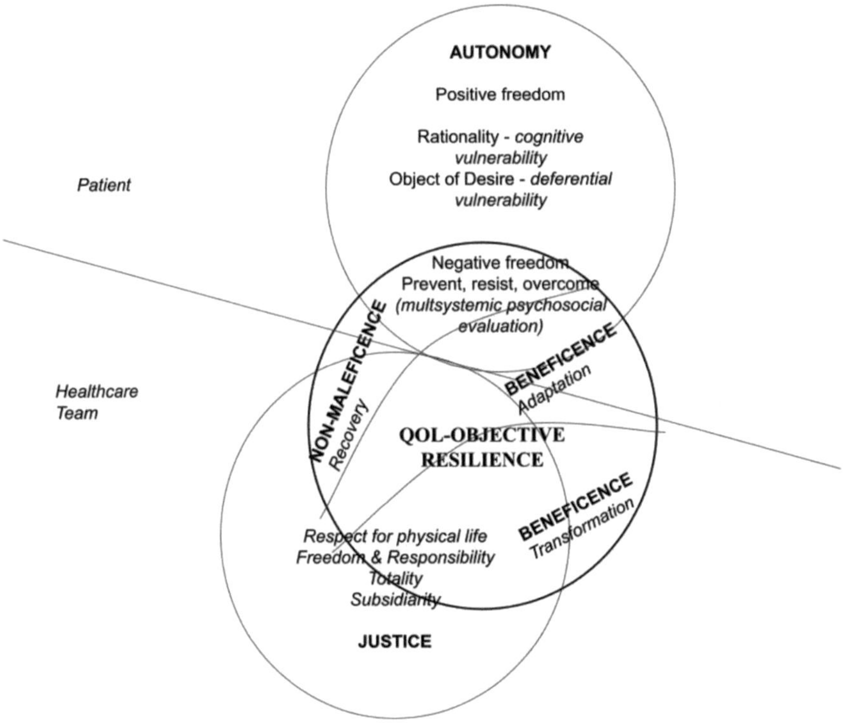

Figure 1.
Bioethical principles in the bioethical deliberation model. Note: QOL-objective resilience is at the center, overlapping with both autonomy of the patient, and justice of the healthcare team. QOL-objective resilience has three levels: Recovery (non-maleficence), adaptation (beneficence), and transformation (beneficence). Autonomy is divided into positive and negative freedom. Some further annotations are included per domain.

According to Honneth's Theory of Recognition [18, 19], essential self-relationships precede autonomous functioning and include self-trust, self-respect, and self-esteem. Although these definitions highlight relevant social values, we believe that it is important to also think about the self-relationships described through the light of a Kantian vision to further highlight a non-movable value—human dignity. The concept of value necessitates a comparison between objects based on a criterion that bestows worth. In Western culture, self-worth adjustment typically occurs through two distinct avenues. The first involves oppressive socialization, where individuals conform to societal standards of beauty, wealth, and intelligence. This process leads to the development of "contingent self-esteem" also named "contingent self-worth, " which depends on meeting specific standards of excellence as outlined by interpersonal or intrapsychic expectations. Alternatively, Kant would argue that self-worth should be based on the unchanging axiom of dignity, which allows no degrees and remains an absolute value despite an individual's failure to meet social standards.

Self-relationships are closely connected to self-worth, which can be understood through the concepts of dignity and respect. Respect, based on Kantian principles, involves treating others as ends rather than means [20] and refraining from abusing someone's vulnerable position in which he or she may be treated as if they were undeserving of dignity—for reasons such as those conveyed by oppressive socialization [21]. Self-respect refers to the ability to treat oneself with dignity and recognize one's absolute value, which cannot be achieved or lost based on external standards or failures. Trust emerges as the expectation that arises from respecting dignity despite flaws, helping to maintain one's worth even when faced with shortcomings. Self-trust is the expectation that one's dignity will be defended and treated with respect by oneself, irrespective of societal expectations or oppressive standards, such as those related to beauty—that oppressively subjugate people's self-recognition of dignity and worth. Self-esteem is a psychological measure of how individuals perceive their relational value and social acceptance by others, as proposed by the sociometer theory [22]. It involves adopting the perspectives and judgments of others, and it fluctuates based on accomplishments and social recognition [23]. It is determined by what is deemed socially valuable or repugnant [24].

The argument goes as follows: if a patient seeks a VCA to increase self-esteem (via diminished social rejection), and so to conceal his or her notion of low self-worth, deferential vulnerability to accept the risks of receiving a transplant is likely to be present. Ways to assess deferential vulnerability are proposed later in the chapter.

2.3 Justice

Justice, as a critical component of transplant success, extends beyond equitable resource allocation to include sensitivity to factors that can bias and impede fair deliberation. We believe transplant success should imply a just bioethical debate that considers objective resilience as the foundation of quality of life and be free of oppressive socialization biases (societal norms, values, and prejudices that may unfairly influence individuals' beliefs, choices, and opportunities [21]). Under oppressive socialization, medical professionals may face external expectations to offer VCA as a solution to patients, even when it may not be the most appropriate or beneficial option. These pressures can stem from societal beliefs regarding beauty standards, the desire to showcase medical advancements, economic considerations, among others. On the other hand, oppressive socialization can perpetuate biases that may unconsciously influence the medical team's perception of patients, potentially leading to unequal treatment, disregard for patient autonomy, or inappropriate candidate selection. It is important to recognize and address these biases to ensure fair and just decision-making processes.

Overall, justice as a component of transplant success requires not only fair resource allocation but also a commitment to promoting objective resilience and ensuring that ethical deliberations are free from oppressive socialization biases.

After operationalizing each principle, we can say that *transplant success in the context of VCA involves a procedure that is autonomously chosen by the patient and fairly allocated by the healthcare team. It aims to effectively promote patient objective resilience, while also addressing the patient's main motivations and facilitating recovery, adaptation, and transformation.*

Based on the proposed definition of transplant success, a process is proposed that seeks to evaluate and promote the conditions for the possibility of transplant success. For this, the bioethical deliberation model has been outlined. This model encompasses an assessment of both the patient's and the healthcare system's capacity, focusing on two dimensions: deliberative *capacity* and *receiver-offering* capacity. By evaluating these aspects, the model aims to ensure a thorough and comprehensive evaluation process that upholds the principles of beneficence, non-maleficence, autonomy, and justice. It seeks to minimize the impact of oppressive socialization biases and promote a fair and ethical approach to decision-making in VCA.

In this chapter, the elements of the bioethical deliberation model are described both for patients and healthcare teams. In addition, methods or tools for the evaluation or exploration of the domains are described or proposed for either the patient or the healthcare teams.

3. Bioethical deliberation model for VCA

In a general sense, the bioethical deliberation model encompasses the steps for evaluation (through the assessment of deliberative capacity and receiver and offering capacity) and the elements for deliberation and design of strategies (third phase) aligned with the criteria that define success in VCA. For the evaluation phase both for the patient and the healthcare team, it addresses the elements and necessary conditions to, in the negative sense, prevent, resist, and cope with flaws in the corresponding dimension and stakeholder. In the positive sense, it explores the elements and necessary conditions to operate based on maxims that correspond to the greatest good sought by each dimension of the model. In this sense, the aim is to *protect* (negative sense) against factors that distort the optimal functioning of the dimension and *promote* (positive sense) the maximum expression of the good sought by the factor.

Next, a more detailed description will be provided regarding the elements and necessary conditions for evaluating the deliberative capacity and receiver and offering capacity in both the negative and positive sense. Subsequently, the dimension or phase of deliberation and design will be discussed (**Figure 2**).

3.1 Deliberative capacity

Deliberative capacity encompasses the principles of autonomy and justice.

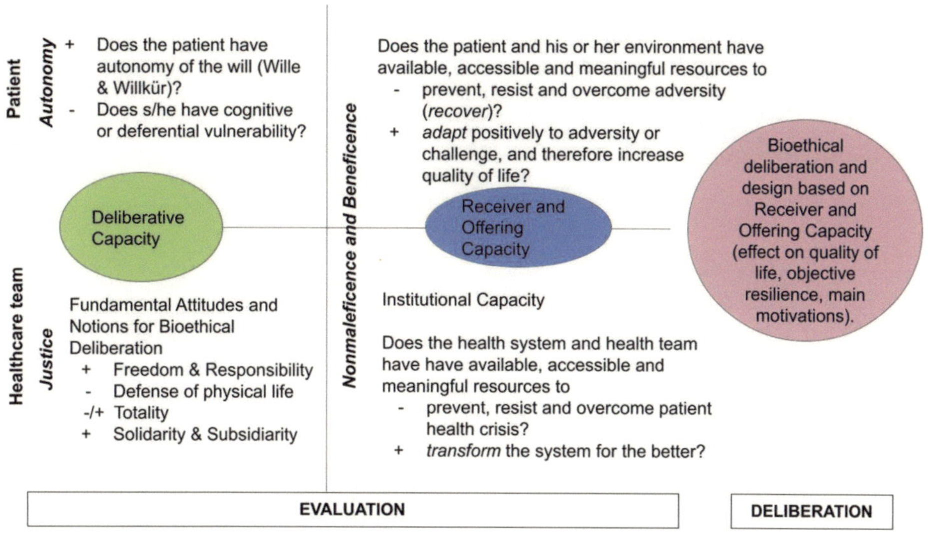

Figure 2.
Bioethical deliberation model for VCA. Note: Bioethical deliberation model. + = positive sense (promote); – = negative sense (protect).

3.1.1 Patient

In relation to the patient, it refers to their ability to autonomously deliberate and choose whether to undergo VCA, taking into account the capacity to prevent, resist, and overcome limitations in their autonomy (negative sense), and to effectively express the will through decision-making capacity, clarity in weighing risks and benefits, among others (positive sense).

The assessment of the patient's deliberative capacity involves comprehensive psychiatric and psychological evaluations aimed at evaluating the autonomy of their will and deferential vulnerability. It is important to recognize the current lack of standardized tools to assess this vulnerability accurately. Therefore, there is an urgent need to develop reliable scales that measure the proposed self-relationships and examine their relationship with autonomy in decision-making. However, as previously described, a qualitative method based on self-relationships is proposed to evaluate deferential vulnerability, which directly impacts decision-making (and consequently compromises consent) and could obstacle treatment adherence. We propose and continue to develop a theoretical framework informed by a Kantian interpretation of Honneth's Recognition Theory [18, 19] (Farías-Yapur, under review), as described in the Autonomy section. This section provides a practical proposal for evaluating self-relationships, which is schematically illustrated in **Figure 3**. It incorporates Honneth's practical self-correlations and interprets them through the notion of Dignity according to Kant, which provides the normative content upon which the practical self-correlations are defined. Furthermore, it is contrasted with the possible expression of the self-relationships in the context of oppressive socialization.

To assess patients' self-relationships and the influence of public perception on their self-worth, we suggest considering some key dimensions. This will primarily be achieved through clinical interviews, where we will explore the presence of self-respect or its absence (evident in shame, self-rejection, etc.) in events where there

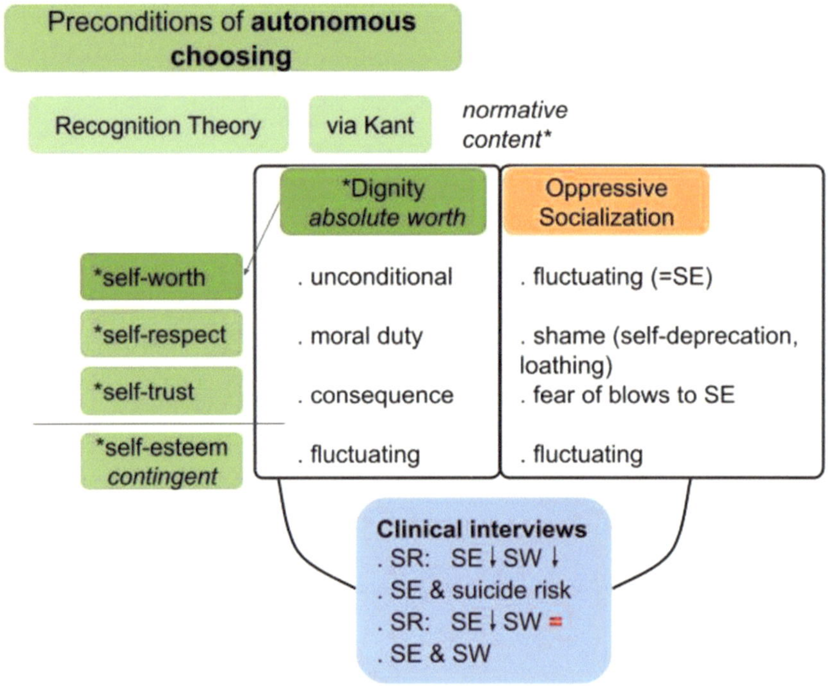

Figure 3.
Evaluating self-relationships. Note: SR = self-respect, SW = self-worth, it is observed that under the context of oppressive socialization, self-esteem determines self-worth, and there is an absence of self-respect, leading to a high presence of shame and probable fear of self-esteem injuries [25]. The key questions proposed, although preliminary and not exhaustive, are briefly shown in blue to guide the clinical interview. We can anticipate that the critical variable is the presence or absence of self-respect.

have been injuries to the patient's self-esteem or in critical situations such as suicidal ideation or attempts. Monitoring shame carefully serves as an important indicator of potential risk factors for depression and suicidality [25, 26], and may also act as a powerful motivator for seeking VCA, such as face transplantation, as a means of restoration [5].

In clinical interviews, there are four complementary thematic axes that focus on specific elements of the patient's discourse, aimed at understanding the functioning of their practical self-relationships and the potential threat of self-esteem to self-worth. The first thematic axis consists of evidence that the deterioration of self-esteem impairs self-worth, indicating an absence of self-respect. The second thematic axis incudes exploring the impact of deteriorating self-esteem on suicide risk (and identifying mechanisms that prevented suicide such as competing ideas, support networks, etc.). It is important to understand the main causes of suicidal ideation and the resources the patient used to prevent it, as this may provide indications of self-respect. It is noteworthy that several patients seeking VCA face-transplantation have a need derived from trauma resulting from unsuccessful suicide attempts. However, it is important to understand the main causes of these attempts and, based on that information, determine whether they are related to the effects of oppressive socialization or responses to significant impairments to their resilience. The third thematic axis is investigating the independence of self-worth from self-esteem. This involves exploring whether the patient's self-worth remains intact despite a decline in self-esteem in various events, potentially due to self-respect. Finally, assessing the presence of self-esteem as a complementary positive self-relationship to self-worth. It is important to note that self-esteem only poses a risk when self-respect is lacking, and it is possible to have a healthy self-esteem and self-worth. Self-esteem, being socially influenced, is related to a sense of transcendence, such as helping other patients prevent risks that led to accidents requiring VCA, among others. As mentioned earlier, throughout this evaluation, special attention should be given to the experience of shame, which is a significant emotional and attitudinal response associated with devaluing self-worth.

The proposed schema suggests conducting a similar assessment of the patient's family to determine whether there is oppressive socialization within the family that causes the patient to perceive a lack of social recognition as an indicator of low dignity. This may result in pressure, albeit well-intentioned, for the patient to undergo an intervention requiring lifelong immunosuppressants.

In addition to measuring autonomy to validate informed consent, it is crucial to delve into the patient's primary motivations that guide their consideration of VCA as a suitable strategy. This comprehensive evaluation aims to uncover their expectations regarding the potential impact of VCA on various dimensions of their objective resilience. Understanding these motivations is paramount, as they shed light on the patient's main objectives and aspirations for a better quality of life. Examining these motivations provides valuable insights into the feasibility of their attainment, alternative approaches to achieving them, potential implications for treatment adherence in the event of failure, and other pertinent considerations that inform the decision-making process. By considering these factors, healthcare professionals can better understand the patient's perspective and tailor the approach to VCA accordingly.

3.1.2 Healthcare team

Regarding the healthcare team, deliberative capacity refers to their ability to engage in ethical deliberation that is just and unbiased, by having the skills to, in a negative sense, prevent, resist, and overcome flaws in their judgment. It involves being sensitive to biases, understanding the critical dimensions of objective resilience, possessing deliberation skills, and adhering to protective principles such as respect for physical life and totality. Additionally, in a positive sense, it entails promoting the skills to deliberate and actively practice justice through the principles of sociability and subsidiarity, freedom and responsibility, and totality.

While psychiatric evaluations have been recommended for team members to ensure their deliberative capacity, in Mexico we propose conducting an evaluation of fundamental attitudes and key concepts for bioethical deliberation to provide evidence-based training. Some key aspects to evaluate include Moral Competence, Moral Teamwork, Moral Action, Notions of objective resilience as multisystemic and as the basement of quality of life, among others.

To assess the state of each of these aspects within the healthcare team, the following instruments are used: the Euro-MCD 2.0 Instrument is utilized to measure participants' perception of their own abilities such as moral sensitivity, analytical skills, virtuous attitude, open dialog, supportive relationships, moral decision-making, and responsible care. As the principles of Personalistic Bioethics are proposed as integral to the practice of justice and subsequent deliberation and design, the agreement with Personalistic principles is also evaluated.

3.2 Receiver and offering capacity

Regarding the dimension of the receiver and offering capacity, concerning the patient's receiver capacity, it is crucial to note that without an environment with accessible and relevant resources available to solve problems or promote individual and social development, their achievement, no matter how motivated the patient may be, will be impossible. In that sense, a significant part of evaluating the patient's receiver capacity goes beyond their individual resources or attitudes, etc., and instead asks about the environment and how it should be for the person to recover and adapt from adversity or to achieve flourishing.

In the negative sense, the evaluation considers the elements and necessary conditions to prevent, resist, and overcome adversities derived from VCA, such as everything required to achieve treatment adherence. This level of resilience corresponds to *recovery* and has an effect on the patient's objective resilience of *non-maleficence*. On the other hand, in a positive sense, the evaluation examines the elements and necessary conditions for positive *adaptation* to the patient's life circumstances with VCA, corresponding to a level of resilience higher than recovery and an effect of VCA on the patient's objective resilience and quality of life of *beneficence*.

3.2.1 Patient

To achieve an increase in objective resilience and quality of life, both at the recovery and adaptation/transformation levels, it is necessary to consider the protective and risk factors present in the multiple systems in which the patient operates. For this purpose, a comprehensive evaluation of the patient's objective resilience involves conducting a multisystemic psychosocial assessment, recognizing that resilience is a complex process that operates within various interconnected systems, including the individual themselves.

While there are existing psychosocial evaluation tools such as the PACT, TERS, and SIPAT instruments [27–30], we supplement their use with clinical interviews guided by a framework developed by Farías-Yapur et al. [6], as these instruments mainly evaluate individual and some microsystem aspects, while neglecting others, such as those specific to developing countries (which is a risk factor for successful patient outcomes). The guide incorporates Bronfenbrenner's Theory of Social Ecology [11], which includes six proposed systems (individual, microsystem, mesosystem, exosystem, macrosystem, and chronosystem), along with Ungar's three resilience process components (availability, accessibility, and meaningfulness of resources necessary for preventing, resisting, and overcoming adversity). An exploratory literature review was conducted, paying special attention to whether the framework and traditional instruments covered psychosocial risk factors that explained failed VCA cases. To include risk factors not reported in the literature and specific to the Mexican context, a semi-structured interview was developed to explore the experiences of patients who had undergone VCA in the corresponding country, in order to understand the obstacles and strategies across the proposed dimensions during their pre and post-surgical treatment.

By utilizing this framework, the evaluation process enables the identification of multisystemic risk and protective factors that impact treatment adherence, a critical behavior for the success of transplantation. A preliminary review of the multisystemic protective and risk factors is shown in **Figure 4**, taken from Farías-Yapur, A. [6].

Table 1 A systemic approach to psychosocial domains of interest in VCA

Desired outcomes: treatment adherence, graft survival positive patient outcomes	What resources should be available at macro-, exo-, meso-, micro-, and individual level? Ungar's multisystemic social-ecological theory	What factors facilitate and hinder access to such necessary resources or their functionality?	What macro-, exo-, meso-, micro-, and individual factors influence how treatment is followed/available resources are used?
	Availability of resources	Accessibility to resources	Treatment implementation
Macrosystem	Legal regulation for VCA (+) Donation culture (graft) (−) No preventive health behaviors	(+) Awareness of VCA (−) Feeling shame of being vulnerable (−) Power structures	(−) Conflicting medicine frameworks (−) Biases in perception of prescription's relevance due to power structures (−) Feeling shame of being vulnerable
Exosystem	Grafts Trained multidisciplinary health team Interconsultation services Formation of assessment, intervention, and follow-up teams Immunosuppressant and other medication	(−) Inefficient bureaucracy (−) Inconsistent or conflicting policies (+) Consistent health insurance policies (−) Difficulty getting medication (−) Difficulty getting to the hospital for follow-ups or emergencies	(−) Conflicting evidence (−) Unavailable research (−) Unknown or rigid procedures for special populations
Cronosystem	What key resources does stability depend on? Consider changing social, economic, and political contexts.		
Mesosystem	Communication channel and coordination between microsystems	(+) Efficient intergroupal communication:health teams, family members, employers, insurance, and financial aid providers (+) Efficient intergroupal communication:health teams, family member employers, insurance, and financial aid providers (+) Communication and arrangement between key microsystem's actors to increase their response capacity to patient needs	(+) Common understanding of the role and importance of the microsystems interconsultation teams, relevant family (+) Common treatment goals, and understanding of particular objectives in relation to main goals (+) Collaboration between microsystem
Cronosystem	What key resources does stability depend on? Consider Ungar's phases of key exosystemic and microsystemic resources.		
Microsystem	Support networks: family, peers, employers, health care team, insurance providers Economic, emotional and practical support Time availability of support networks (family members) to assist the patient with adhering to treatment	(−) Networks' saturation of resource use: time money physical space, attention, etc. (+) Sustainable support strategies (burnout) (+) Family cohesion and adaptability	(+) Trust in doctor-patient relationship (+) Common treatment goals (+) Coherence and common sense of treatment (+) Understanding of most relevant aspects of treatment
Cronosystem	What key resources does stability depend on? What key resources does stability depend on? Consider key resources "reserves" depletion in high stress and chronic situation (burnout)		
Individual	Economic resources (with reserve), adequate housing, time availability, support networks and above systems' resources Cognitive and decision-making capacities Cognitive and decision-making capacities	(+) Health insurance (−) Mood and personality disorders (−) Neuropsychological disorders (−) Internalization of oppressive socialization (low self-worth self-respect and self-esteem)	(+) Coherence and common sense of treatment (−) Unrealistic expectations of transplant outcomes (+) Congruence between objective transplant outcome expectations and patients main goals (−) Vulnerability as a threat to self-esteem (+) High self-efficacy, problem-solving coping style (+) Self-care health behaviors (−) Use of alcohol, nicotine (−) Mood disorder (depression)
	Cronosystem What key resources does stability depend on? Consider high stress and chronic situations.		

(+): The factor increases availability and accessibility to resources, or meaningfulness of the treatment. (−): The factor obstacles availability and accessibility to resources, or meaningfulness of the treatment

Curr Transpl Rep

Springer

Figure 4.
Exploratory review of risk and protective factors to promote treatment adherence as a critical variable for recovery. Note: As shown, in this case, the review and interviews were conducted with previous VCA patients to identify risk and protective factors for achieving treatment adherence. However, the dependent (desired) variable can be any other variable, and the reflection can be approached with the same orientation and classification.

Based on the developed classification mode, the factors of interest described in the literature, the risk factors that explain transplant failures, the semi-structured interviews conducted with arm transplant patients in Mexico, as well as the factors that are not described but correspond to proposed dimensions, a multisystemic psychosocial assessment guide was developed, where the factors to be evaluated corresponding to each proposed dimension in Farías-Yapur et al. [6] are presented in the form of sub-items and questions.

In addition to the multisystemic approach, administering quality of life measures is helpful to estimate subjective notions of well-being, as well as expectations for its improvement. Useful measures include the SF-36 QoL [9] scale, as well as the WHOQOL [8]. Based on information gathered by the aforementioned assessments, a simplified representation of the effect of VCA on critical domains is desirable, such that it helps improve bioethical deliberation regarding patient candidacy, as well as to better tailor specific domains to improve patient candidacy. An example of this (**Figure 5**) could involve a visual representation where the height of the blue line informs about the potential effect of VCA on the current objective resilience of the patient. This visualization provides a clearer understanding of the impact of VCA on the patient's overall well-being and aids in decision-making processes.

3.2.2 Healthcare team

Regarding the offering capacity of the healthcare team, in a negative sense, we inquire about the necessary elements and conditions to prevent, resist, and overcome

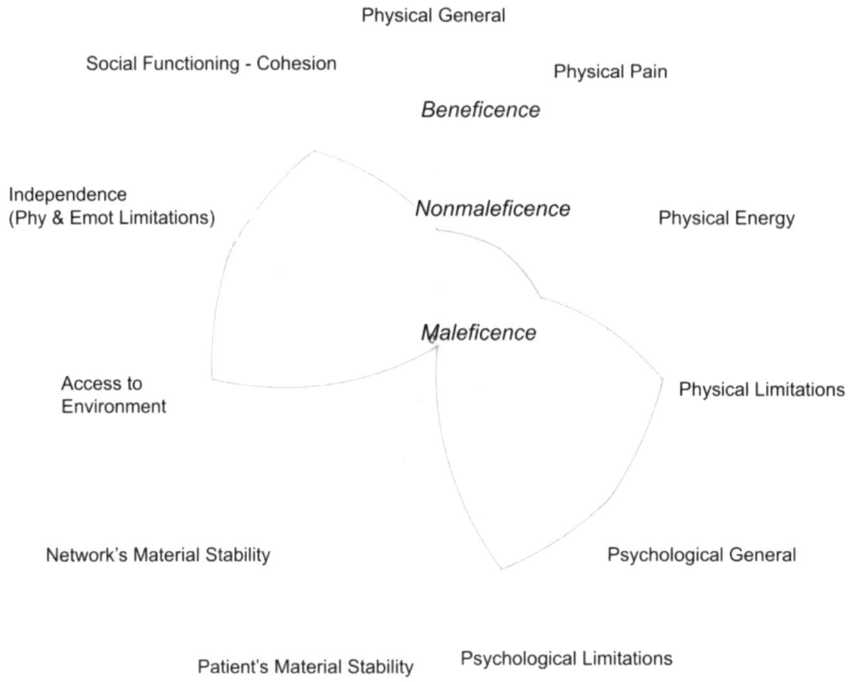

Figure 5.
Estimation of the effect of VCA on objective resilience (not real data). Note: Estimated effects are based on the assumption of receiving VCA with current objective resilience.

obstacles to patient treatment adherence (recovery, non-maleficence). In a positive sense, we explore the elements and conditions required to achieve the transformation of the system and environment that influence the overall resilience of the population (which corresponds to the highest level of impact and increase in multisystemic resilience).

As part of the systems with which the patient interacts from a multisystemic perspective, we have the microsystem of the healthcare team itself, whose interaction with the other relevant systems constitutes the mesosystem. The proposed approach involves examining whether the system has access to the necessary and accessible resources to successfully carry out VCA and create conditions that enable patients to overcome adversities.

It has been reported that the quality of collaboration within the healthcare team is a crucial factor that predicts patient success [31]. According to Babiker et al. [32], "an effective team is one where the team members, including the patients, communicate with each other, as well as merging their observations, expertise, and decision-making responsibilities to optimize patients' care." The general institutional capacity of the team can be assessed, and a useful tool for this is the Clinical Sustainability Assessment Tool [33]. In addition to assessing institutional capacity on its own, factors related to the internal functioning of the microsystem in terms of communication, mesosystemic communication (with the patient and support networks), and the integration of information from all involved parties must be evaluated.

Based on the multisystemic psychosocial assessment guide and the preliminary guide to support the evaluation of institutional capacity developed by the Bioethics Team of the VCA Subcommittee (Anneke Farías Yapur, Juan Manuel

Palomares, Marieli de los Ríos Uriarte, Elvira Llaca García) the following domains are proposed for evaluation: 1) Comprehensive treatment, common goals, updated information; 2) Communication with the patient; 3) Integration of all involved services, including the patient.

In the context of comprehensive treatment, effective communication, and integration of all involved services, participants are presented with a series of statements to gauge their agreement levels. These statements cover various aspects, such as common goals, shared understanding of success for each patient, established processes for case analysis, and addressing doubts from all stakeholders. Furthermore, communication with the patient emphasizes clear dissemination of relevant information, thorough explanation of treatment implications involving consultative services, ensuring clarity about the next steps, understanding the purpose of each treatment element and phase, identifying and resolving obstacles to treatment adherence, and actively involving the patient in the treatment design. Additionally, the integration of all involved services aimed to establish clear short-term and long-term goals, define transplant success in alignment with bioethical principles, ensure a comprehensive understanding of the quality of life among patients, families, and physicians, establish and evolve transplant goals over time, and communicate both short-term and long-term objectives.

Based on the results obtained, training programs are designed for the subcommittee, and improvements are designed and implemented in the patient-family-healthcare team mesosystem.

3.3 Bioethical deliberation and subsequent design

Finally, in the phase of bioethical deliberation and design of the next steps, the entire healthcare team is involved, and the results obtained during the previous phase are considered. Deliberation and the design of the next steps are based on the personalistic principles of respect for physical life, the principle of totality, solidarity and subsidiarity, and freedom and responsibility.

One crucial aspect of this deliberation is identifying any maleficence effects that may arise in specific domains of the patient's resilience. These red flags serve as indicators to explore alternative designs that, at the very least, do not worsen the patient's objective resilience. For instance, the economic impact of VCA on personal finances is a significant consideration. If it is determined that the financial burden of VCA is negative, proceeding with may not be feasible, unless sustainability is guaranteed. Therefore, it is essential to ensure that all dimensions of objective resilience predict a minimum effect of non-maleficence, although it is important to note that non-maleficence alone would not justify the pursuit of VCA, given the promise to enhance the patient's quality of life.

To illustrate and simplify data, we represent effects on objective resilience domains in terms of an ordinal scale to denote beneficence if the line touches the outer circle, non-maleficence if it stays in the middle circle, and maleficence if it touches the center, as shown in **Figure 5**.

To foster resilience and mitigate potential negative impacts, strategies that promote the former should be incorporated into the design. This may include interventions such as healthcare inclusion and work inclusion, which can have positive effects on the patient's overall well-being and adherence to treatment sustainability. Collaborating with professionals such as social workers, psychologists, legal experts, and occupational therapists is crucial in designing and implementing resilience-promoting interventions. Occupational therapists, in particular, play a vital role in helping individuals regain and enhance their functional abilities, independence, and overall well-being, making their involvement essential in the VCA process.

3.4 Case example

The evaluation process begins with a thorough assessment of the patient's autonomy and deferential vulnerability through clinical and psychiatric interviews, as described in the corresponding section. A comprehensive multisystemic evaluation is then carried out to estimate the potential effect of the transplant on the patient's objective resilience and quality of life. This evaluation encompasses various domains, as summarized in **Table 1**, and takes into account the estimated effects on objective resilience as depicted in **Figure 5**. **Table 1** presents the main domains with key information regarding the presence of risk factors or contraindications. This information allows us to quickly review the patient's current systems' resilience and the expected impact of VCA on patient objective resilience.

Preliminary deliberations with the subcommittee are guided by fundamental principles such as respect for physical life, totality, subsidiarity, and freedom and responsibility. Respect for physical life serves as a boundary when considering interventions. Totality emphasizes that any intervention will affect the entirety of the person's life domains. The principle of subsidiarity is crucial as it calls for a generous attitude, especially in developing countries and when working with vulnerable populations. Finally, freedom and responsibility highlight the notion of being free yet accountable for all aspects of life.

Aligned with these principles, deliberations are held to define the next steps after discussing the current risk factors that predict harm as an effect of VCA. Strategies are proposed to improve patient candidacy and the effect of VCA on the patient's

Main Motivations: elements, hypothetical failure situation	**themes**
Decision-making capacity (mental examination, psychiatric disorders, vulnerability of deference-autonomy).	No contraindications.
Material (financial situation, hospital debt, social insurance).	Risk factor.
Support network + (availability of the network, type of support, sustainable timeframe).	Available, practical, emotional, economic, medium-term (risk factor if there is no job reintegration or stable support program - long term).
Support network - (obstacles to coherence and meaning of treatment, network exhaustion, long-term support, financial sustainability).	Risk factor.
Linkage between microsystems (patient-family, healthcare team, clear and timely communication).	Risk factor.
Quality of Life (SF, WHOQOL).	Determining factor: *theme*
Estimated Impact on Objective Resilience.	Beneficial for most dimensions, but a risk factor for individual material stability and support network.

Table 1.
Summary of a preliminary multisystemic psychosocial evaluation.

objective resilience and quality of life. For example, enlisting the patient for job security. As the patient's candidacy evaluation progresses, ongoing evaluations and training sessions are provided to the healthcare team and VCA subcommittee, tailored to the Mexican context. Additionally, continuous assessment of the capacity to offer VCA is conducted, allowing for iterative improvements in processes, with the ultimate goal of achieving transformation and optimizing outcomes.

It is expected that after systematically following the proposed bioethical deliberation model, the conclusion would be that the patient has autonomously deliberated with knowledge and understanding of the risks and benefits, without a determining pressure to conform to social expectations, and that they desire VCA as a practical strategy to achieve their goals. In addition to having the capacity to weigh and decide, in the case of a successful transplant, it is expected that the patient actively engages to enhance their understanding and deliberative capacity, and they co-create the therapeutic strategy with the healthcare team. On the other hand, a successful VCA case also entails that the individual, as well as their environment, has availability and access to critical resources to 1) prevent, resist, and overcome adversities related to VCA treatment (thus achieving non-maleficence *recovery*) and 2) positively *adapt* to their life circumstances with VCA (resulting in a beneficial effect). Additionally, a successful VCA case implies that the healthcare system has the necessary means to ensure non-maleficence and recovery in the patient's objective resilience and to guarantee beneficence and adaptation in the patient's objective resilience and quality of life. Finally, it also signifies that the healthcare system has the necessary mechanisms to improve and transform the system and the conditions that improve the multisystemic resilience of the population.

4. Discussion

In the realm of VCA, ethical deliberation plays a pivotal role in safeguarding the well-being of patients and guiding healthcare systems. To address the intricate considerations surrounding VCA and foster informed and ethical decision-making processes, the proposed bioethical deliberation model represents a significant advancement.

Built upon the fundamental principles of beneficence, non-maleficence, autonomy, and justice, as well as the principles of Personalist Bioethics, the model is crafted to align with the bedrock of ethical healthcare practices. By focusing on three key dimensions, namely deliberative capacity, reception-offering capacity, and the deliberation & subsequent design phase, the model provides a robust framework for evaluating and promoting the readiness and suitability of both the patient and the healthcare system for VCA.

At the heart of the model lies the recognition of objective resilience as a critical determinant of success and a catalyst for patient well-being. Objective resilience encapsulates an individual's capacity to navigate, withstand, and triumph over adversities, thereby enhancing their overall quality of life. By adopting a multisystemic approach to assess objective resilience, the model enables a comprehensive evaluation that takes into account the interconnectedness of various systems contributing to an individual's resilience.

In conclusion, the proposed bioethical deliberation model offers a structured and comprehensive approach to evaluate VCA procedures, facilitate ethical decision-making, and elevate patient care and treatment outcomes. By thoughtfully considering the critical variables that define beneficence, non-maleficence, autonomy, and justice, this model provides valuable insights into navigating the intricacies of the ethical landscape surrounding VCA. Ultimately, the model serves as a guiding compass for enhancing the well-being of both patients and healthcare systems, exemplifying the ethical aspirations of the VCA field.

Author details

Anneke Farías-Yapur
Interdisciplinary Center for Bioethics, Panamerican University, Mexico City, Mexico

*Address all correspondence to: 0184151@up.edu.mx

References

[1] Liu X, Langsdon S, Holloway W, Xu S, Tang Q, Xu Y, et al. The ethics of facial Allotransplantation: A systematic review. Plastic and Reconstructive Surgery. Global Open. 2019;**7**(10):e2425. DOI: 10.1097/GOX.0000000000002425

[2] Shanmugarajah K, Hettiaratchy S, Butler PEM. Facial transplantation. Current Opinion in Otolaryngology & Head and Neck Surgery. 2012;**20**(4):291-297. DOI: 10.1097/moo.0b013e3283552cc5

[3] Alexander AJ, Alam DS, Gullane PJ, Lengelé BG, Adamson PA. Arguing the ethics of facial transplantation. Archives of. Facial Plastic Surgery. 2010;**12**(1):60-63. DOI: 10.1001/archfacial.2009.106

[4] Madani H, Hettiaratchy S, Clarke A, Butler PE. Immunosuppression in an emerging field of plastic reconstructive surgery: Composite tissue allotransplantation. Journal of Plastic, Reconstructive & Aesthetic Surgery. 2008;**61**(3):245-249. DOI: 10.1016/j.bjps.2007.08.011

[5] Theodorakopoulou E, Meghji S, Pafitanis G, Mason KA. A review of the world's published face transplant cases: Ethical perspectives. Scars, Burns & Healing. 2017;**3**:1-10. DOI: 10.1177/2059513117694402

[6] Farías-Yapur A, Iglesias M, González-Chávez A, Cantú-Quintanilla G. A multisystemic approach to psychosocial evaluations of vascularized composite allotransplantation candidates. Current Transplantation Reports. 2020. DOI: 10.1007/s40472-020-00293-z

[7] Alberti FB, Hall S, Pow R, Sreenan N, & Ridley M. About Face: A Blueprint for Sustainable Face Transplant Policy and Practice. 2022. Available from: https://aboutfaceyork.com/wp-content/uploads/2022/05/AboutFace_PolicyLabReport-3.pdf; https://aboutfaceyork.com/resource/a-blueprint-for-sustainable-face-transplant-policy-and-practice/

[8] World Health Organization. The World Health Organization Quality of Life (WHOQOL) - BREF, 2012 Revision. Geneva: World Health Organization; 2004. Available from: https://apps.who.int/iris/handle/10665/77773

[9] Ware JE, Sherbourne CD. The MOS 36-item short-form health survey (SF-36). I. Conceptual framework and item selection. Medical Care. 1992;**30**:473-483

[10] Ungar M, editor. Multisystemic Resilience: Adaptation and Transformation in Contexts of Change. Online edn. New York: Oxford Academic; 18 Mar 2021. DOI: 10.1093/oso/9780190095888.001.0001. [Accessed: 13 July 2023]

[11] Bronfenbrenner U. The Ecology of Human Development: Experiments by Nature and Design. JSTOR, Harvard University Press; 1979. DOI: 10.2307/j.ctv26071r6 [Accessed: 13 July 2023]

[12] Pietrzykowski T, Smilowska K. The reality of informed consent: Empirical studies on patient comprehension—Systematic review. Trials. 2021;**22**(1):60-63. DOI: 10.1186/s13063-020-04969-w

[13] Beauchamp TL. Informed consent: its history, meaning, and present challenges. Camb Q Healthc Ethics. Oct 2011;**20**(4):515-523. DOI: 10.1017/S0963180111000259. PMID: 21843382

[14] Dandry T, Catalano J. Legal, Ethical and Political Issues in Nursing. Philadelphia, PA: Davis; 1993

[15] Davis AJ, Aroskar MA. Ethical Dilemmas and Nursing Practice. 2nd ed. East Norwalk, CT: Prentice-Hall; 1983

[16] Kipnis K. Vulnerability in research subjects: A bioethical taxonomy. In: National Bioethics Advisory Commission, editor. Ethical and Policy Issues in Research Involving Human Participants. Bethesda: National Bioethics Advisory Commission; 2001. pp. G1-G13 http://www.aapcho.org/wp/wp-content/uploads/2012/02/Kipnis-VulnerabilityinResearchSubjects.pdf

[17] Melton GB, Petrila J, Poythress NG, Slobogin C. Psychological Evaluation for the Courts: A Handbook for Mental Health Professionals and Lawyers. 2nd ed. New York: Guilford Press; 1997

[18] Honneth A. The Struggle for Recognition. Cambridge, England: Polity Press; 1995

[19] Honneth A. The Struggle for Recognition: The Moral Grammar of Social Conflicts. Cambridge, MA: MIT Press; 1996

[20] Massey SJ. Is self-respect a moral or a psychological concept? Ethics. 1983;**93**(2):246-261. DOI: 10.1086/292432

[21] Benson P. Autonomy and oppressive socialization. Social Theory and Practice. 1991;**17**(3):385-408. DOI: 10.5840/soctheorpract199117330

[22] Leary MR. Sociometer theory. In: Van Lange PAM, Kruglanski AW, Higgins ET editor. Handbook of Theories of Social Psychology. London: Sage Publications Ltd.; 2012. pp. 151-159. DOI :10.4135/9781446249222.n33

[23] Crocker J, Knight KM. Contingencies of self-worth. Current Directions in Psychological Science. 2005;**14**(4):200-203. DOI: 10.1111/j.0963-7214.2005.00364.x

[24] Pereira G. Más allá del liberalismo: El enfoque de las capacidades y la justicia social crítica. Tópicos, Revista de Filosofía. 2016;**51**:105-130 Recuperado de http://topicosojs.up.edu.mx/ojs/index.php/topicos/article/view/759/741

[25] Hastings ME, Northman LM, Tangney JP. Shame, guilt, and suicide. In: Suicide Science. Boston, MA: Springer; 2002. DOI: 10.1007/0-306-47233-3_6

[26] Weingarden H, Renshaw KD, Wilhelm S, Tangney JP, DiMauro J. Anxiety and shame as risk factors for depression, suicidality, and functional impairment in body dysmorphic disorder and obsessive compulsive disorder. The Journal of Nervous and Mental Disease. 2016;**204**(11):832-839. DOI: 10.1097/nmd.0000000000000498

[27] Jowsey-Gregoire S, Kumnig M. Standardizing psychosocial assessment for vascularized composite allotransplantation. Current Opinion in Organ Transplantation. 2016;**21**(5):530-535. DOI: 10.1097/mot.0000000000000351

[28] Maldonado JR, Dubois HC, David EE, Sher Y, Lolak S, Dyal J, et al. The Stanford integrated psychosocial assessment for transplantation (SIPAT): A new tool for the psychosocial evaluation of pretransplant candidates. Psychosomatics. 2012;**53**(2):123-132. DOI: 10.1016/j.psym.2011.12.012

[29] Olbrisch ME, Levenson J, Hamer R. The PACT: A rating scale for the study of clinical decision-making in psychosocial screening of organ transplant candidates. Clinical Transplants. 1989;**3**:164-169

[30] Twillman RK, Manetto C, Wellisch DK, Wolcott DL. The transplant evaluation rating scale. Psychosomatics. 1993;**34**(2):144-153. DOI: 10.1016/s0033-3182(93)71905-2

[31] Schmutz JB, Meier LL, Manser T. How effective is teamwork really? The relationship between teamwork and performance in healthcare teams: A systematic review and meta-analysis. BMJ Open. 2019;**9**(9):e028280. DOI: 10.1136/bmjopen-2018-028280

[32] Babiker A, El Husseini M, Al Nemri A, Al Frayh A, Al Juryyan N, Faki MO, et al. Health care professional development: Working as a team to improve patient care. Sudanese Journal of Paediatrics. 2014;**14**(2):9-16

[33] Malone S, Prewitt K, Hackett R, Lin JC, McKay V, Walsh-Bailey C, et al. The clinical sustainability assessment tool: Measuring organizational capacity to promote sustainability in healthcare. Implementation Science Communications. 2021;**2**(1):77. DOI: 10.1186/s43058-021-00181-2

Chapter 7

Allogeneic Islet Transplantation and Future

Shinichi Matsumoto, Sadaki Asari, Yoshihide Nanno and Takumi Fukumoto

Abstract

Pancreatic islets contain beta cells which produce insulin based on the blood glucose levels resulting in tight control of blood glucose levels. In type 1 diabetic patients, most of the beta cells are destroyed, therefore, pharmaceutical insulin injection is mandatory to avoid diabetes-related illness and death. Even with recent advanced insulin therapy, hypoglycemia is a critical limiting factor to control blood glucose levels. There is no doubt that hypoglycemia can be fatal. Allogeneic islet transplantation can prevent severe hypoglycemia and provide excellent blood glucose control. On the other hand, allograft donor shortage is the major issue. To overcome donor shortage, xenograft has been used and shown safety and efficacy. Recently stem-cell-derived beta cells are clinically applied. In this chapter, the history and current status of allogenic islet transplantation and future scope are described.

Keywords: islet transplantation, allograft, type 1 diabetes, hypoglycemia, xenogeneic islet transplantation

1. Introduction

Type 1 diabetes is a devastating disease due to its acute and chronic complications. Acute complications include hyperglycemic ketoacidosis and hypoglycemic attack, and both complications can be life-threatening. Chronic complications include nephropathy which leads to the necessity of hemodialysis, retinopathy which leads to blindness, and neuropathy which causes necrosis of the legs and the necessity of amputation.

Intensive insulin therapy is the gold standard for type 1 diabetic patients, which significantly reduces the risk of chronic complications and mortality rates [1]. However, intensive insulin therapy was associated with weight gain and a threefold increased risk for hypoglycemia [1], and hypoglycemia is a limiting factor for intensive insulin therapy [2]. Indeed, 4–10% of type 1 diabetic patients died due to hypoglycemia [3].

Since the cause of type 1 diabetes is destruction of insulin-secreting beta cells, beta cell replacement therapies are curative treatments [4]. Beta cell replacement therapies include the pancreas and islet transplantation. Allogeneic islet transplantation can prevent severe hypoglycemia and provide excellent glycemic control. On the other hand, donor shortage is a major issue. In this chapter, the current situation of allogenic islet transplantation and potential resolution of donor shortage is described.

2. History of allogeneic islet transplantation

The idea of isolating islets of Langerhans using collagenase was originally published in 1965 [5]. With this method, Guinea pig pancreas was minced and digested with collagenase resulting in obtaining isolated islets. Washington University group introduced the intra-ductal injection method to improve the islet isolation method [6]. In fact, the Washington University group demonstrated that the first successful reversal of diabetes by islet isolation using diabetic rat model [7]. An important innovation was reported by the Stanford University group. They inject collagenase into pancreatic duct resulting in adequate islets for transplantation from a single donor using a canine model [8]. This method enables to initiate the first clinical trial of allogeneic islet transplantation at the University of Minnesota.

The first clinical trial of allogeneic islet transplantation was performed in 1970s' at the University of Minnesota (**Table 1**), however, did not achieve improving metabolic control [9, 10, 21]. The first successful allogeneic islet transplantation into type 1 diabetic patients was reported by Zurich University group (**Table 1**) [10]. In this first successful case, the patient received simultaneous kidney and islet transplantation, and islets were transplanted into a spleen. The patient achieved insulin independence 8 months after transplantation and maintained it for 10 months. Notably, the age of the donor was 2 years old, and islets from young donor can be suitable for islet transplantation. However, the patient suffered

Year	Events	Authors	Reference
1965	Development of islet isolation with collagenase	Moskalewski S	[5]
1972	First successful islet transplantation in rodent	Ballinger WF, Lacy PE	[7]
1977	First clinical islet transplantation	Najarian JS, Sutherland DER Matas et al.	[9]
1980	First successful islet transplantation	Largiader F, Kolb E, Binswanger U	[10]
1988	Development of automated method for islet isolation	Ricordi C, Lacy PE, Finke EH, Olack BJ, Scharp DW	[11]
1990	First series of successful islet transplantation	Tzakis AG, Ricordi C, Alejandro R, et al.	[12]
1994	First clinical islet xenotransplantation	Groth CG, Korsgren O, Tibell A, et al.	[13]
2000	First clinical encapsulated islet xenotransplantation without immunosuppression	Elliott RB, Escobar L, Garkavenko O, et al.	[14]
2000	Edmonton protocol	Shapiro AM, Lakey JR, Ryan EA, et al.	[15]
2005	First successful living donor islet transplantation	Matsumoto S, Okitsu T, Iwanaga Y, et al.	[16]

Year	Events	Authors	Reference
2006	First series of successful islet transplantation from non-heart-beating donor	Matsumoto S, Okitsu T, Iwanaga Y, et al.	[17]
2016	Phase 3 clinical trial of islet alone transplantation	Hering BJ, Clarke W, Bridge ND, et al.	[18]
2021	Phase 3 clinical trial of islet after kidney transplantation	Markmann JF, Rickels MR, Eggerman TL, et al.	[19]
2021	Stem cell-derived pancreatic endoderm cell implantation	Shapiro AJM, Thompson D, Donner TW, et al.	[20]

Table 1.
History of islet transplantation.

rejection and died after one month of rejection. Intrasplenic pancreatic islets were detected in the necrotic specimens.

A turning point for clinical islet transplantation was the introduction of the automated method of pancreas dissociation by Camillo Ricordi (**Table 1**) [11]. This method consists of a mechanically enhanced enzymatic digestion based on a dissociation-filter chamber (Ricordi chamber) allowing islets freed from gland to be removed promptly from the system to avoid over-digestion while preserving cluster integrity. This method is called Ricordi method. Washington University group performed a clinical trial of islet transplantation for three type 1 diabetic patient using the Ricordi method, however, all patients lost graft function [22].

The first series of sustained insulin independence following islet transplantation with Ricordi method was achieved for the patients after excision of liver and pancreas, and transplant of allogeneic liver and islet from the same cadaveric donors (**Table 1**) [12]. In these cases, 6 out of 10 patients achieved insulin independence for 5 to more than 16 months [23]. The group also conducted the combined liver-islet allograft transplantation for 4 patients with cirrhosis and diabetes, and the combined kidney and islet transplantation for 7 patients with end-stage renal disease due to type 1 diabetes [23]. None of the patients achieved insulin independence although islet graft function was confirmed.

In 1990, Washington University group reported the first case of insulin independence after purified allogeneic islet transplantation for the treatment of type 1 diabetes [24]. Since then insulin independence after islet transplantation was reported by other centers.

In 1994, Justus-Liebig University reported 30% insulin independence after allogenic islet transplantation [25], in 1997, the San Raffaele Institute reported 45% insulin independence after allogeneic islet transplantation [26].

The Islet Transplant Registry reported the outcomes of 267 allogeneic islet transplantation cases from several centers from 1990 until 2001 [27]. Insulin independence rate was 12.4% for periods greater than one week and 8.2% for greater than one year.

3. Edmonton protocol of allogeneic islet transplantation (new era)

In 2000, the University of Alberta group published that 7 out of 7 type 1 diabetic patients became insulin independent one year after allogeneic islet transplantation (**Table 1**) [15]. Their islet transplantation protocol was named

Protocol	Induction	Maintenance
Edmonton protocol	Daclizumab	Sirolimus, low dose tacrolimus
Islet alone transplantation	Anti-thymocyte globulin for the first transplant Basiliximab for the subsequent transplants	Sirolimus, low dose tacrolimus
Islet after kidney transplantation	Anti-thymocyte globulin (ATG) for the first transplant Basiliximab for the subsequent transplants and in a single case of suspected sensitivity to ATG	Calcineurin-based immunosuppression regimen used for the renal transplant. Up to 10 mg of prednisone

Table 2.
Immunosuppression protocol for allogeneic islet transplantation.

the Edmonton protocol. In their clinical trial, patients received two or three islet transplantations to achieve target doses. The average islet doses were 11,547 islet equivalent (IEQ)/body weight (kg). Immunosuppression was initiated immediately before transplantation. Sirolimus and low-dose tacrolimus were used for maintenance immunosuppression. In addition, Daclizumab was given intravenously every 14 days for a total of five doses (**Table 2**). Isolated islets were not cultured and transplanted as soon as possible.

International trial of the Edmonton protocol for islet transplantation was conducted [28]. The primary endpoint was insulin independence with adequate glycemic control 1 year after the final transplantation. Several secondary endpoints including insulin independence with adequate glycemic control throughout follow-up; improved values for levels of glycated hemoglobin, the mean amplitude of glycemic excursions, and basal and stimulated blood C-peptide levels, and a reduction in the need for insulin. Nine islet transplantation centers participated. The success rate of achieving primary endpoint varies among the 9 centers. The success rates were 100% in one center, 40–80% in five centers and 0% in three centers. They concluded with the Edmonton protocol of islet transplantation, insulin independence is usually not sustainable, however, persistent islet function even without insulin independence provides protection from severe hypoglycemia and improved levels of glycated hemoglobin.

In 2005, five year follow-up after islet transplantation was published by the University of Alberta group [29]. They concluded islet transplantation can relieve glucose instability and problems with hypoglycemia. C-peptide secretion was maintained in the majority of subjects for up to 5 years, although most reverted to using insulin. Since then, islet transplantation is considered a treatment to stabilize blood glucose levels and avoid hypoglycemia, not insulin independence.

4. Phase 3 trial of allogeneic islet transplantation

4.1 Islet alone transplantation

In the United States, allogeneic islet cells are regulated by the FDA as a drug, and expected to be approved under the biological license [18]. In 2016, a license-enabling multicenter phase 3 clinical trial was reported (**Table 1**) [27]. For this study, well-defined islet products were manufactured under Current Good Manufacturing Practices and Current Good Tissue Practices [30]. The collaborative islet transplantation (CIT) consortium created the protocol for manufacturing islet products. Under CIT protocol, 324 pancreata were processed, and 170 products (52.5%) met the product release criteria. Patients received 75 of 170 successfully manufactured islet products were transplanted. For immunosuppression, they used anti-thymocyte globulin and etanercept for induction for the first transplant, with basiliximab replacing anti-thymocyte globulin at subsequent transplant (**Table 2**). Sirolimus and low-dose tacrolimus were used for maintenance immunosuppression. Twenty-two patients received one transplantation, 25 patients received two transplantation and one patient received three transplantation. The primary endpoint was the achievement of HbA1c < 7% and freedom from severe hypoglycemic events from day 28 to day 365 after the first transplantation. The primary endpoint was successfully met by 87.5% of patients, and it was concluded that islet transplantation should be considered for patients with type 1 diabetic patients and impaired awareness of hypoglycemia in whom other less invasive current treatments have been ineffective in preventing severe hypoglycemic events.

In 2018, improved health-related quality of life in phase 3 islet transplantation in type 1 diabetes complicated by severe hypoglycemia was reported [31]. The Diabetes Distress Scale (DDS), the hypoglycemic Fear Survey (HFS), the Short Form 36 Health Survey (SF-36), and the EuroQoL 5 Dimensions (EQ-5D) were applied before and after islet transplantation at days 75, 365, and 730. DDS measured emotional burden, physician-related distress, regimen-related distress, interpersonal distress, and total score. HFS measured hypoglycemic avoidance behavior, worry about hypoglycemia, and total score.

After transplantation, all items of both DDS and HFS significantly improved in every measure point. This indicated allogeneic islet transplantation can improve the QOL related to diabetes and hypoglycemia from day 75 to day 730.

SF-36 measured physical functioning scale, role physical scale, bodily pain scale, general health scale, vitality scale, social functioning scale, physical component summary (PSC), and mental component summary (MSC) (**Table 3**).

Measures	Visit	Mean (SD)	P value
PSC	Baseline	47.52 (8.77)	–
	Day 75	49.97 (8.05)	N.S.
	Day 365	52.52 (7.69)	<0.0001
	Day 730	52.44 (9.06)	0.0004
MCS	Baseline	49.23 (10.48)	–
	Day 75	53.03 (9.65)	0.0081
	Day 365	51.86 (8.94)	N.S.
	Day 730	54.40 (7.28)	N.S.
Physical Functioning scale	Baseline	50.62 (8.04)	–
	Day 75	53.30 (6.58)	0.0034
	Day 365	53.67 (7.17)	0.0005
	Day 730	52.29 (10.26)	N.S.
Role Physical scale	Baseline	45.69 (10.57)	–
	Day 75	49.17 (9.72)	0.0008
	Day 365	51.70 (7.53)	<0.0001
	Day 730	52.67 (9.04)	<0.0001
Bodily Pain scale	Baseline	50.52 (10.04)	–
	Day 75	49.96 (10.97)	N.S.
	Day 365	52.72 (8.24)	N.S.
	Day 730	53.22 (10.19)	N.S.

Measures	Visit	Mean (SD)	P value
General Health scale	Baseline	44.31 (12.42)	–
	Day 75	50.19 (10.45)	<0.0001
	Day 365	51.57 (9.92)	<0.0001
	Day 730	51.60 (11.57)	0.0064
Vitality scale	Baseline	48.81 (10.94)	–
	Day 75	54.67 (8.92)	0.0001
	Day 365	53.38 (8.53)	0.0029
	Day 730	55.38 (10.62)	0.0015
Social Functioning scale	Baseline	46.99 (10.87)	–
	Day 75	49.38 (9.72)	N.S.
	Day 365	50.98 (8.24)	N.S.
	Day 730	51.70 (10.25)	N.S.
Role Emotional scale	Baseline	48.02 (10.25)	–
	Day 75	51.58 (8.72)	N.S.
	Day 365	50.82 (8.43)	0.0090
	Day 730	52.11 (7.49)	N.S.
Mental Health scale	Baseline	51.54 (9.27)	–
	Day 75	53.83 (9.09)	N.S.
	Day 365	53.69 (8.20)	N.S.
	Day 730	54.30 (8.26)	N.S.

Table 3.
Summary of SF 36 [31].

After transplantation, at day 365 and 730, PCS was significantly improved, and at day 75, MCS was significantly improved. In each item, the physical functioning scale was significantly improved after transplantation at day 75 and 365, role physical scale, general health scale, and vitality scale, were significantly improved at all points, role emotional scale was significantly improved after transplantation at day 365. On the other hand, there was no significant change in the bodily pain scale, social functioning scale, and mental health scale.

EuroQoL measured health preference weight, usual activities, anxiety/depression, mobility, pain/discomfort, self-care, and a visual analog scale of overall health (VAS) (**Table 4**). EuroQoL demonstrated that after transplantation at 365 day VAS was significantly improved, and at 730 VAS and usual activities were significantly improved.

Measures	Visit	Mean (SD) or N no problems (%)	P value
VAS	Baseline	74.13 (14.66)	–
	Day 75	79.06 (15.97)	N.S.
	Day 365	82.86 (14.46)	<0.0001
	Day 730	85.74 (15.36)	<0.0001
Health preference weight	Baseline	0.87 (0.12)	–
	Day 75	0.86 (0.15)	N.S.
	Day 365	0.86 (0.15)	N.S.
	Day 730	0.88 (0.18)	N.S.
Usual activities	Baseline	32 (68.09%)	–
	Day 75	35 (74.47%)	N.S.
	Day 365	33 (78.57%)	N.S.
	Day 730	27 (84.38%)	0.0143

Measures	Visit	Mean (SD) or N no problems (%)	P value
Anxiety/depression	Baseline	32 (68.09%)	–
	Day 75	34 (72.34%)	N.S.
	Day 365	29 (69.05%)	N.S.
	Day 730	23 (71.88%)	N.S.
Mobility	Baseline	38 (80.85%)	–
	Day 75	40 (85.11%)	N.S.
	Day 365	34 (82.93%)	N.S.
	Day 730	26 (81.25%)	N.S.
Pain/discomfort	Baseline	25 (53.19%)	–
	Day 75	27 (57.45%)	N.S.
	Day 365	24 (57.14%)	N.S.
	Day 730	22 (68.75%)	N.S.
Self-Care	Baseline	45 (95.74%)	–
	Day 75	46 (97.87%)	N.S.
	Day 365	39 (92.86%)	N.S.
	Day 730	29 (90.63%)	N.S.

Table 4.
Summary of EuroQOL [31].

However, all other measurements had no significant improvements. Allogeneic islet transplantation dramatically improved hypoglycemia-related QOL.

4.2 Islet after kidney transplantation

In 2021, a phase 3 trial of human islets after kidney transplantation in type 1 diabetes was reported (**Table 1**) [19]. This was an open-label, single-arm study involving subjects with type 1 diabetes who had previously received kidney transplantation conducted at 10 centers in North America. The primary endpoint was achieving HbA1c level equal to or less than 6.5%, or reduction in HbA1c of at least 1 point from baseline to day 365, and freedom from severe hypoglycemic events from day 28 to day 365 after the initial islet transplant. For immunosuppression, induction immunosuppression consisted of rabbit anti-thymocyte globulin (ATG) and etanercept for the first transplant, with basiliximab replacing ATG for subsequent transplant and in a single case of suspected sensitivity to ATG (**Table 2**). The calcineurin-based maintenance immunosuppression regimen used for the renal transplant was continued after the islet transplant. Up to 10 mg of prednisone was allowed as part of maintenance immunosuppression.

Twenty-four patients who experienced kidney transplantation received allogeneic islet transplantation. Elven patients received single transplantation, 11 patients received two transplantations, and 2 patients received 3 transplantations. After islet transplantation at 365 days, 15 patients (62.5%) met primary endpoints. They also measured DDS and HFS before and after islet transplantation at day 75, 365, 730, and 1095. Both DDS and HFS demonstrated improved QOL after islet transplantation in type 1 diabetic patients who previously received kidney transplantation at all time points. This study also indicated that islet transplantation is effective treatment for patients with type 1 diabetes and unstable glucose control despite intensive insulin treatment, supporting the indication for islet transplantation in the post-renal transplant setting.

More general QOL was assessed with Euro QOL Visual Analog Scale (VAS). EuroQOL VAS from baseline to day 75, day 365, day 730, and day 1095 following islet transplantation were statistically analyzed. The P-values at day 75 were 0.1016 at day 75, 0.0002 at day 365, 0.0952 at day 730, and 0.0327 at day 1095.

In 2022, long-term outcomes with islet-alone transplantation and islet-after-kidney transplantation for type 1 diabetes in the clinical islet transplantation consortium were reported [32]. Islet alone (n = 48) and islet-after-kidney (n = 24) transplant recipients were followed up to 8 years after allogeneic islet transplantation. The primary endpoint is duration of sustained islet allograft function as determined by evidence from MMTT of c-peptide production at each anniversary of the final transplant. A c-peptide level greater than or equal to 0.3 ng/mL at 0, 60, or 90 minutes will be considered evidence of islet allograft function.

Among them, 26 islet patients and 8 patients for islet-after-kidney patients completed long-term follow-up with islet graft function, 15 and 7 withdrew from follow-up with islet graft function, and 7 and 9 experienced graft failure, respectively.

5. Efforts to improve the efficacy of allogeneic islet transplantation

Phase 3 clinical trial of allogeneic islet transplantation demonstrated the benefit of the islet transplantation, on the other hand, the success rate of production was 52.5%. Improving the success rate is critically important to utilize precious human donor pancreas.

Baylor Research Institute group demonstrated seven consecutive successful clinical islet isolations using the pancreatic ductal injection technique [33]. The average islet yield was 588,566 ± 64,319 islet equivalent (IEQ), and 6 islet products were implanted into 3 type 1 diabetic patients. All three patients achieved insulin free. They demonstrated that ductal injection immediately after pancreas procurement could enhance the delivery of collagenase resulting in the high success rate of islet isolation [34]. The group also analyzed the 100 human islet isolation, then revealed that in addition to the ductal injection, pancreas procurement by the islet isolation team, two-layer pancreas preservation, and short cold ischemic period had a significant impact to improve the success rate of islet isolation [35]. Among them, the two-layer pancreas preservation was created by Dr. Takashi Kawamura and Dr. Yoshikazu Kuroda (**Figure 1**) [36]. The two-layer method consists of an organ preservation solution and perfluorocarbon. During the preservation by the two-layer method, oxygen is continuously supplied through the perfluorocarbon, and the pancreas can be oxygenized. This method provided the longest preservation period before whole pancreas transplantation using canine model [37] and high islet yield [38]. The first clinical trial of the two-layer preservation before pancreas transplantation and islet isolation was both conducted at the University of Minnesota [39, 40]. Oxygen charged two-layer method was developed to eliminate bringing an oxygen tank for continuous oxygenation [41]. The two-layer pancreas preservation was used for clinical islet transplantation using a non-heart-beating donor (**Table 1**) [17] and the first successful living donor islet transplantation (**Table 1**) [16].

Even improving the efficacy of islet transplantation is important, as long as donor source is human, it is not possible to treat all type 1 diabetic patients who need islet transplantation.

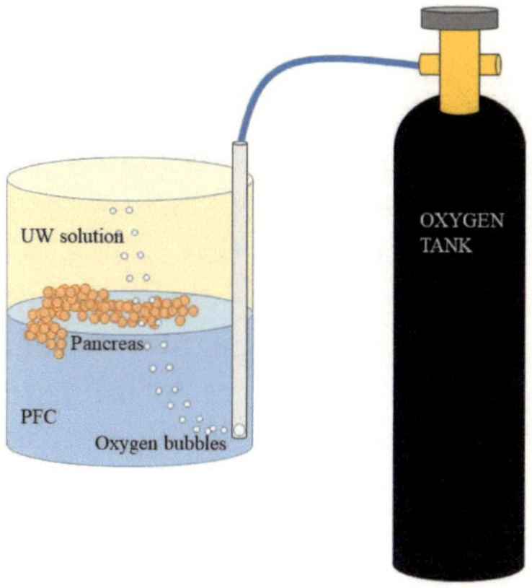

Figure 1.
Two-layer preservation method consists of perfluorocarbon (PFC) and organ preservation solution (for example University of Wisconsin (UW) solution). PFC is unsolvable in the water therefore, PFC and organ preservation solution clearly created the two-layer. The procured pancreas locates between the PFC and organ preservation solution. Oxygen has been provided to PFC for the original two-layer method. For oxygen static charged two-layer method, before using the two-layer preservation method, PFC was fully oxygenated. Fully oxygenated PFC could reserve adequate oxygen concentration for up to 18 hours. During preservation by the two-layer method, pancreas has been oxygenated and maintained high energy status. The two-layer pancreas preservation enabled the longest preservation period before canine whole pancreas transplantation and improved islet yield after human islet isolation.

6. Overcome the issue of donor shortage

6.1 Clinical porcine islet xenotransplantation

In 1994, transplantation of porcine islet-like cell clusters (ICCs) was implanted into 10 insulin-dependent diabetic kidney transplant patients (**Table 1**) [13]. Among the 10 patients, 8 patients received ICCs into the portal vein and the other two patients received ICCs under the kidney capsule. Four patients who received ICCs into portal vein secreted porcine C-peptide for 200 to 400 days. A biopsy was conducted on one patient who received ICCs under kidney capsule, and ICCs with positive insulin and glucagon stains were detected. On the other hand, insulin reduction was not achieved.

In 2000, two cases of encapsulated neonatal porcine islet transplantation were reported (**Table 1**) [14]. The first patient was a 41-year-old male who had type 1 diabetes for 18 years and required 50 units insulin per day. He received total of 13,000,000 IEQ encapsulated porcine islets. The second patient was a 39-year-old female who had type 1 diabetes for 24 years. She required 49 units of insulin per day. She received kidney transplantation two years before this islet transplantation; therefore. She took maintenance immunosuppression with cyclosporine, azothiaprine, and prednisone. She received 930,000 IEQ-encapsulated porcine islets. Both patients experienced a significant reduction in frequency of severe hypoglycemic reactions. Porcine C-peptide had been detected over 14 months, and improved HbA1c and 8–40% reduction of insulin were confirmed until 27 months post-transplantation.

More than 9 years after transplantation, the first patient was followed. Oral glucose tolerance test revealed positive porcine insulin. Laparoscopic biopsy demonstrated that the alginate capsule included insulin and glucagon-positive cells [42].

In 2005, twelve adolescent diabetic patients received neonatal porcine islet combined with porcine Sertoli cell transplantation using a subcutaneous device. Eleven patients received second transplantation and 4 patients received third transplantation. At 4 years, half of the patients achieved reduction of insulin doses. Notably, two patients achieved insulin independence [43]. The same group reported long-term follow-up study outcomes of 21 type 1 diabetic patients [44]. The median time post-transplantation was 5.7 years. More than half of the patients reduced insulin doses by more than 30% compared with pre-transplantation. Before transplantation 14 patients had chronic complications of diabetes including neuropathy (n = 5) evidenced by abnormal speed of nervous conduction, non-proliferative diabetic retinopathy (n = 5), and microalbuminuria (n = 8). At the follow-up, only two patients had chronic complications. No patients had neuropathy, 1 patient had retinopathy and 2 patients had microalbuminuria.

In 2011, Wang et al. reported that 22 patients received neonatal porcine islets in the hepatic artery [45]. The first 14 patients were treated with cyclosporine, mycophenolate mofetil (MMF), and prednisolone, the following 2 patients were treated with cyclosporine and MMF, and the next 6 patients were treated with OKT. The first 14 patients required less insulin and improved HbA1c after transplantation. In the 2 subsequent patients did not have any metabolic change and porcine C-peptide was negative. The last 6 patients reduced insulin requirements, and HbA1c was normalized 3 months after the transplantation.

In 2011, Matsumoto et al. reported that 14 patients in received encapsulated neonatal porcine islets in the abdominal cavity without immunosuppressive drugs in New Zealand [46]. Patients received 5000 (n = 4), 10,000 (n = 4), 15,000 (n = 4), and 20,000 (n = 2) IEQ/kg islets. There were no apparent differences among the groups. Patients experienced reduction of unaware hypoglycemia and minimal change in HbA1c and insulin doses one year after transplantation. In 2016, the same group reported 8 patients who received encapsulated neonatal porcine islets in the abdominal cavity without immunosuppressive drug in Argentina [47]. Four patients received 10,000 IEQ/kg and the other 4 patients received 20,000 IEQ/kg. All patients improved HbA1c, and high dose group demonstrated a significant reduction in the number of unaware hypoglycemia. They also demonstrated no zoonosis after 5–7 years of islet xenotransplantation [48]. Recently, they reported 21 patients' opinions who received encapsulated neonatal porcine islet transplantation after approximately 10 years [49]. Importantly, no patients suffered zoonosis, and no patients suffered cancer. Compared with pre-transplantation, the majority of patients still improved glycemic control, diabetic management, and reduced severe hypoglycemic events and hyperglycemia required hospitalization even after 10 years of transplantation. All patients considered this treatment adequate and majority of patients wanted to recommend this treatment to the other patients and desired to receive booster transplantation.

6.2 Stem cell-derived beta cell transplantation in clinic

In 2021, stem cell-derived pancreatic endoderm cell transplantation was reported (**Table 1**) [20]. Stem cell-derived pancreatic endoderm cells within the device were transplanted into 17 type 1 diabetic patients. Since the device has no immune protective property, the patients received immunosuppressive drugs. The induction immunosuppression was anti-thymocyte globulin up to 6 mg/kg iv over 5 days, TNF alpha blocking etanercept 50 mg iv pre-implant followed 25 mg subcutaneous x 3 doses after transplant. Maintenance immunosuppression was tacrolimus (target 10–12 ng/mL for the first 3 months; 7-9 ng/mL there-after) and mycophenolate mofetil up to 2 g per day as tolerated.

Primary efficacy endpoint was C-peptide measurements. A total of 6/17 subjects (35.3%) demonstrated stimulated C-peptide at varying time points. Adverse events were related to side effects of immunosuppressive drugs (33.7%) followed by surgical procedures (27.9%).

7. Conclusions

Allogeneic islet transplantation has become the standard therapy for unstable type 1 diabetic patients for avoiding severe hypoglycemia. Considering a large number of type 1 diabetic patients, donor shortage is an issue for allogeneic islet transplantation. To overcome the donor shortage, xenogeneic islet transplantation had been conducted for more than 10 years, and recently stem cell-derived pancreatic endoderm cell transplantation began. With advanced technology, we wish type 1 diabetes will become a curable disease.

Acknowledgements

The authors thank Japan IDDM network for the financial support.

Conflict of interest

Shinichi Matsumoto is a chief scientific officer at Otsuka Pharmaceutical Factory Inc. and an adviser at PorMedTec Inc.

Author details

Shinichi Matsumoto*, Sadaki Asari, Yoshihide Nanno and Takumi Fukumoto
Department of Hepatobiliary Pancreatic Surgery, Kobe University, Kobe, Japan

*Address all correspondence to: shinichi41@mac.com

References

[1] Nathan DM. Realizing the long-term promise of insulin therapy: The DCCT/EDIC study. Diabetologia. 2021;**64**:1049-1058. DOI: 10.1007/s00125-021-05397-4

[2] Cryer PE. Glycemic goals in diabetes: Trade-off between control and iatrogenic hypoglycemia. Diabetes. 2014;**63**:2188-2195. DOI: 10.2337/db14-0059

[3] Cryer PE. Severe hypoglycemia predicts mortality in diabetes. Diabetes Care. 2021;**35**:1814-1816. DOI: 10.2337/dc12-0749

[4] Matsumoto S, Shimoda M. Current situation of clinical islet transplantation from allogeneic toward xenogeneic. Journal of Diabetes. 2020;**12**:733-741. DOI: 10.1111/1753-0407.13041

[5] Moskalewski S. Isolation and culture of the islets of Langerhans of the guinea pig. General and Comparative Endocrinology. 1965;**44**:342-353

[6] Lacy PE, Kostianovsky M. Method for the isolation of intact islets of Langerhans from the rat pancreas. Diabetes. 1967;**16**:218-223

[7] Ballinger WF, Lacy PE. Transplantation of intact pancreatic islets in rats. Surgery. 1972;**72**:175-186

[8] Horiguchi A, Merrell RC. Preparation of viable islet cells from dogs by a new method. Diabetes. 1981;**30**:455-458

[9] Najarian JS, Sutherland DE, Matas AJ, et al. Human islet transplantation: A preliminary report. Transplantation Proceedings. 1977;**9**:233-236

[10] Largiader F, Kolb E, Binswanger U. A long-term functioning human pancreatic islet allotransplant. Transplantation. 1980;**29**:76-77

[11] Ricordi C, Lacy PE, Finke EH, Olack BJ, Scharp DW. Automated method for islet isolation of human pancreatic islets. Diabetes. 1988;**31**:421-426

[12] Tzakis AG, Ricordi C, Alejandro R, et al. Pancreatic islet transplantation after upper abdominal exenteraion and liver replacement. Lancet. 1990;**336**:402-405

[13] Groth CG, Korsgren O, Tibell A, et al. Transplantation of porcine fetal pancreas to diabetic patients. Lancet. 1994;**344**:1402-1404. DOI: 10.1016/s0140-6736(94)90570-3

[14] Elliott RB, Escobar L, Garkavenko O, et al. No evidence of infection with porcine endogenous retrovirus in recipients of encapsulated porcine islet xenografts. Cell Transplantation. 2000;**9**:895-901

[15] Shapiro AM, Lakey JR, Ryan EA, et al. Islet transplantation in seven patients with type 1 diabetes mellitus using a glucocorticoid-free immunosuppression regimen. The New England Journal of Medicine. 2000;**343**:230-238. DOI: 10.1056/NEJM200007273430401

[16] Matsumoto S, Okitsu T, Iwanaga Y, et al. Insulin independence after living-donor distal pancreatectomy and islet allotransplantation. Lancet. 2005;**365**:1642-1644. DOI: 10.1016/s0140-6736(05)66383-0

[17] Matsumoto S, Okitsu T, Iwanaga Y, et al. Successful islet transplantation from nonheartbeating donor pancreata using modified Ricordi islet isolation method. Transplantation. 2006;**82**:460-465. DOI: 10.1097/01.tp.0000231710.37981.64

[18] Hering BJ, Clarke W, Bridge ND, et al. Phase 3 trial of transplantation of human islets in type 1 diabetes complicated by severe hypoglycemia. Diabetes Care. 2016;**39**:1230-1240. DOI: 10.2337/dc15-1988

[19] Markmann JF, Rickels MR, Eggerman TL, et al. Phase 3 trial of human islet-after-kidney transplantation in type 1 diabetes. American Journal of Transplantation. 2021;**21**:1477-1492

[20] Shapiro AJM, Thompson D, Donner TW, et al. Insulin expression and C-peptide in type 1 diabetes subjects implanted with stem cell-derived pancreatic endoderm cells in an encapsulation device. Cell Reports Medicine. 2021;**2**:100466

[21] Sutherland DE, Matas AJ, Goetz FC, Najarian JS. Transplantation of dispersed pancreatic islet tissue in humans: Autografts and allografts. Diabetes. 1980;**29**(Supple 1):31-44

[22] Scharp D, Lacy P, Ricordi C, et al. Human islet transplantation in patients with type 1 diabetes. Transplantation Proceedings. 1989;**21**:2744-2745

[23] Ricordi C, Tzakis AG, Carroll PB, et al. Human islet isolation and allotransplantation in 22 consecutive cases. Transplantation. 1992;**53**:407-414

[24] Scharp DW, Lacy PE, Santiago JV, et al. Insulin independence after islet transplantation into type 1 diabetic patient. Diabetes. 1990;**39**:515-518

[25] Hering BJ, Bretzel RG, Hopt UT, et al. New protocol toward prevention of early human islet allograft failure. Transplantation Proceedings. 1994;**26**:570-571

[26] Secchi A, Socci C, Maffi P, et al. Islet transplantation in IDDM patients. Diabetologia. 1997;**40**:225-231

[27] Brendel MD, Hering BJ, Schultz AO, Bretzel RG. International Islet Transplant Registry. Germany: Giessen; 2013

[28] Shapiro AM, Ricordi C, Hering BJ, et al. International trial of the Edmonton protocol for islet transplantation. The New England Journal of Medicine. 2006;**355**:1313-1330. DOI: 10.1056/NEJMoa061267

[29] Ryan EA, Peter BW, Senior PA, et al. Five-year follow-up after clinical islet transplantation. Diabetes. 2005;**54**:2060-2069. DOI: 10.2337/diabetes.54.7.2060

[30] Ricordi C, Goldstein J, Balamurugan AN, et al. National institute of health-sponsored clinical islet transplantation consortium phase 3 trial: Manufacture of a complex cellular product at eight processing facilities. Diabetes. 2016;**65**:3418-3428. DOI: 10.2337/db16-0234

[31] Foster ED, Bridges ND, Feurer ID, et al. Improved health-related quality of life in a phase 3 islet transplantation trial in type 1 diabetes complicated by severe hypoglycemia. Diabetes Care. 2018;**41**:1001-1008. DOI: doi.org/10.2337/dc17-1779

[32] Rickels M, Eggerman TL, Bayman L, et al. Long-term outcomes with islet-alone and islet-after-kidney transplantation for type 1 diabetes in the clinical islet transplantation. Diabetes Care. 2022;**45**:2967-2975

[33] Matsumoto S, Noguchi H, Shimoda M, et al. Seven consecutive successful clinical islet isolations with pancreatic ductal injection. Cell Transplantation. 2010;**19**:291-297. DOI: 10.3727/096368909X481773

[34] Shimoda M, Itoh T, Sugimoto K, et al. Improvement of collagenase distribution with the ductal preservation for human

islet isolation. Islets. 2012;**4**:130-137. DOI: 10.4161/isl.19255

[35] Takita M, Matsumoto S, Noguchi H, et al. One hundred human pancreatic islet isolations at Baylor research institute. Proceedings (Baylor University Medical Center). 2010;**23**:341-348. DOI: 10.1080/08998280.2010.11928648

[36] Kawamura T, Kuroda Y, Suzuki Y, et al. Seventy-two-hour preservation of the canine pancreas by the two-layer (Euro-Collins' solution/perfluorochemical) cold storage method. Transplantation. 1989;**47**:776-778. DOI: 10.1097/00007890-198905000-00005

[37] Fujino Y, Kuroda Y, Suzuki Y, et al. Preservation of canine pancreas for 96 hours by a modified two-layer (UW solution/perfluorocarbon) cold storage method. Transplantation. 1991;**51**:1133-1135. DOI: 10.1097/00007890-199105000-00044

[38] Matsumoto S, Rigley TH, Reems JA, Kuroda Y, Stevens RB. Improved islet yields from Macaca nemestrina and marginal human pancreata after two-layer method preservation and endogenous trypsin inhibition. American Journal of Transplantation. 2003;**3**:53-56. DOI: 10.1034/j.1600-6143.2003.30110.x

[39] Matsumoto S, Kandaswamy R, Sutherland DER, et al. Clinical application of the two-layer (University of Wisconsin solution/perfluorochemical plus O2) method of pancreas preservation before transplantation. Transplantation. 2000;**70**:771-774. DOI: 10.1097/00007890-200009150-00010

[40] Hering BJ, Kandaswamy R, Harmon JV, et al. Transplantation of cultures islets from two-layer preserved pancreas in type 1 diabetes with anti-CD3 antibody. American Journal of Transplantation. 2004;**4**:390-401. DOI: 10.1046/j.1600-6143.2003.00351.x

[41] Matsumoto S, Rigley TH, Qualley SA, Kuroda Y, Reems JA, Stevens RB. Efficacy of the oxygen-charged static two-layer method for short-term pancreas preservation and islet isolation from nonhuman primate and human pancreata. Cell Transplantation. 2002;**11**:769-777

[42] Elliott RB, Escobar L, Tan PLJ, et al. Live encapsulated porcine islets from a type 1 diabetic patient 9.5 yr after xenotransplantation. Xenotransplantation. 2007;**14**:157-161

[43] Valdés-González RA, Dorantes LM, Garibay GN, et al. Xenotransplantation of porcine neonatal islets of Langerhans and Sertoli cells: A 4-year study. European Journal of Endocrinology. 2005;**153**:419-427

[44] Valdes-Gonzalez R, Rodriguez-Ventura AL, White DJ, et al. Long-term follow-up of patients with type 1 diabetes transplanted with neonatal pig islets. Clinical and Experimental Immunology. 2010;**162**:537-542

[45] Wang W, Mo Z, Ye B, Hu P, Liu S, Yi S. A clinical trial of xenotransplantation of neonatal pig islets for diabetic patients. Journal of Central South University (Med Sci). 2011;**36**:1134-1140

[46] Matsumoto S, Tan P, Baker J, et al. Clinical porcine islet xenotransplantation under comprehensive regulation. Transplantation Proceedings. 2014;**46**:1992-1995

[47] Matsumoto S, Abalovich A, Wechsler C, et al. Clinical benefit of islet xenotransplantation for the treatment

of type 1 diabetes. eBioMedicine. 2016;**12**:255-262

[48] Matsumoto S, Wynyard S, Giovannangelo M, et al. Long-term follow-up for the microbiological safety of clinical microencapsulated neonatal porcine islet transplantation. Xenotransplantation. 2020;**27**:e12631

[49] Matsumoto S, Abalovich A, Wynyard S, Carulla ME, Abalovich D. Patients' opinions 10 years after receiving encapsulated porcine islet xenotransplantation without immunosuppression. Xenotransplantation. 2023;**2023**:e12798

Section 3

Particulate Allograft

Chapter 8

Particulate Allografts (DFDBA) Combined with Platelet Concentrate: An Effective Combination for Sinus Lifts and Post-Extraction Bone Grafting

Adnane Wardani and Laurence Evrard

Abstract

Alveolar bone resorption after tooth extraction can lead to considerable loss of bone volume, which can complicate dental implant planning. To limit this bone loss, immediate post-extraction bone grafting is recommended, while maxillary sinus grafting may be necessary in cases of insufficient sub-sinusal bone height. The use of a combination of particulate Demineralized Freeze-Dried Bone Allograft (DFDBA) and platelet concentrates, such as Platelet-Rich-Fibrin (PRF), has shown promising results in alveolar bone preservation after teeth extractions, as well as in sinus bone grafts (sinus lifts). We conducted several studies, both clinical and histomorphological, to find out if the use of this combination of biomaterials could lead to good bone quantity and quality, and be suitable for implants. Following the results of our studies, the use of particulate DFDBA combined with PRF, whether for alveolar bone preservation after dental extractions or sinus lifts, appears to be an effective technique to maintain or recreate bone volume for dental implant placement. Moreover, histomorphometric study shows a good quality and a good maturity of bone gained with this technique.

Keywords: bone graft, DFDBA, sinus lift, platelet concentrate, socket healing, post-extraction bone grafting

1. Introduction

Bone resorption of the maxilla related to tooth loss: The alveolar bone resorption that occurs after tooth extraction is a gradual, inevitable, and irreversible physiological phenomenon. According to studies, this resorption leads to a loss of bone height and thickness of up to 40% and 60%, respectively. The maximum resorption occurs within 3 months to 1 year after extraction, with two-thirds occurring in the first 3 months [1–3].

In the region of single-rooted teeth, resorption occurs mainly in a horizontal direction, while in the region of multi-rooted teeth, it predominantly occurs vertically

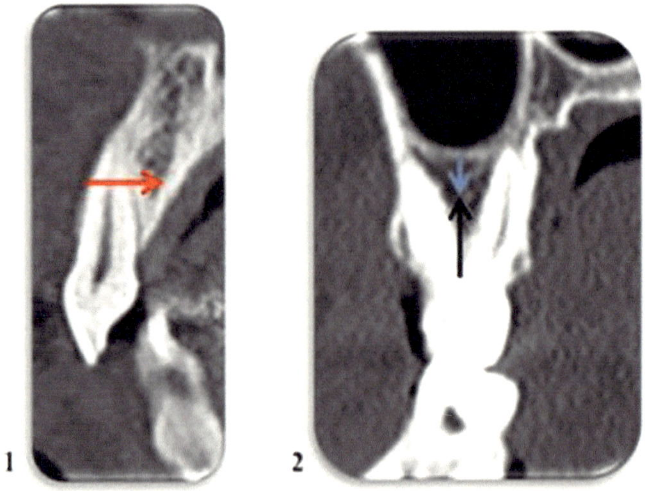

Figure 1.
Single-rooted tooth (1): Bone resorption with a predominant horizontal direction (red arrow). In multi-rooted teeth (2), resorption mainly occurs in a vertical direction, both in the lower level of bone (black arrow) and in the upper level due to pneumatization of the maxillary sinuses resulting from the loss of root support (blue arrow).

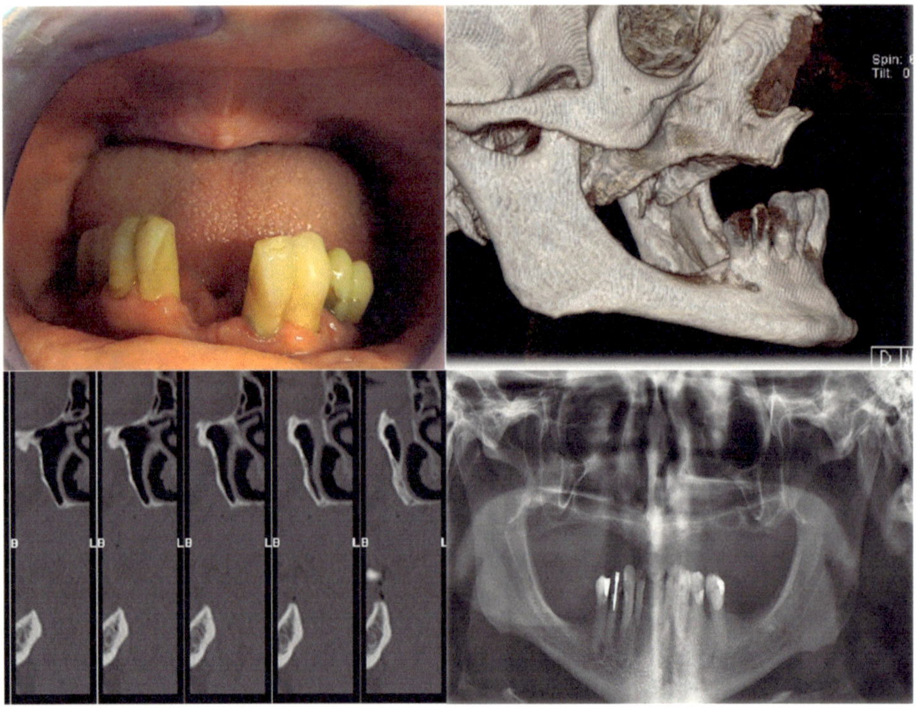

Figure 2.
Clinical view, panoramic radiograph, and CT scan: Centripetal resorption of the upper alveolar crest, resulting in an anteroposterior displacement of the upper crest relative to the lower crest and an inverted maxillary relationship in the direction of an Angle class III.

(**Figure 1**) [1–3]. In the posterior part of the maxilla, this bone resorption is accompanied by a centrifugal pneumatization of the maxillary sinuses that increases with age [4]. The result of this phenomenon is a significant reduction in residual sub-sinus bone height, which may compromise implant placement in this area.

In a retrospective study of 248 edentulous patients, it was observed that less than half of the maxillae of patients over 65 years old have a bone height greater than or equal to 6 mm [4]. Post-extractional resorption can lead to a situation of bone volume loss that may compromise the implant treatment plan. Moreover, in some cases, it results in a modification of the relationships between the bone ridges due to centripetal resorption in the upper maxilla (**Figure 2**), which leads to an unfavorable situation in terms of biomechanics and esthetics.

It has been shown that post-extraction bone volume loss results from two phenomena: loss of the fasciculated bone [2, 3] and colonization of the upper third of the dental alveolus by connective tissue which has the effect of reducing the available space for bone healing [2–4]. There is currently a consensus on the need to perform post-extraction bone filling immediately after extractions to achieve the most optimal bone preservation [1–3, 5, 6], in order to minimize the bone loss that follows dental extractions and to ensure the best possible bone conditions for patient implant rehabilitation. When there is insufficient sub-sinus bone height, it is necessary to resort to a maxillary sinus graft prior to implant placement in this area [7, 8].

2. Techniques used in oral surgery to avoid post-extraction bone volume loss or increase sub-sinus bone volume

Alveolar ridge preservation and maxillary sinus graft techniques are based on filling respectively the empty alveolus or the space between the sinus floor and the Schneider membrane with biocompatible material, with or without adjuncts, with or without a covering membrane.

2.1 Biomaterials used in oral surgery

Biomaterials used in oral surgery are classified into two categories: Natural origin biomaterials and synthetic origin biomaterials.

2.1.1 Synthetic origin biomaterials

Synthetic origin biomaterials include tricalcium phosphate, hydroxyapatites, biphasic ceramics, bioactive glasses, and polymers [9]. Tricalcium phosphates (ßTCP) $Ca3(PO4)2$ are produced by heating a mixture of calcium phosphate powder and naphthalene to over a thousand degrees and under pressure, which, after sublimation, leaves a porous structure that is responsible for the material's osteoconductive properties. Porous hydroxyapatite $Ca10(PO4)6(OH)2$ is obtained by the thermal transformation of calcium carbonate. Chemically, this calcium phosphate is the closest to biological apatite crystals. Several porosities are available. The higher the porosity, the better the osteoconduction. Biphasic ceramics (BCP) comprise a combination of hydroxyapatite and tricalcium phosphate in varying proportions, allowing the qualities of both materials to be combined, particularly to obtain adequate resorption and mechanical properties. Bioactive glasses, $SiO2P2O5CaONaO$, are materials known as “bioactive.” This “bioactivity” would be due to surface reactions of the bioactive glass and ionic exchanges with biological fluids. The os/bioactive glass bond would be made through a layer of amorphous silica gel that exerts a chemotactic effect on osteoblasts. Polymers, notably polymethylmethacrylate (PMMA), have excellent biocompatibility.

2.1.2 Natural biomaterials natural include xenogeneic bone, natural coral, and allogenic bone

Xenogeneic bone (xenograft) is most commonly derived from pigs or cows. Inorganic bovine bone retains a bone spatial structure, giving it osteoconductive properties. These products are presented in a lyophilized form [9, 10]. Natural coral is composed of 99% calcium carbonate. After thermal treatment, it retains a porous structure that gives it osteoinductive properties [9, 10]. Allogeneic bone substitutes are produced from femoral head bone taken from fresh human cadavers. Compared to autogenous bone, they have the advantage of not requiring bone harvesting from the patient (as autogenous bone harvesting carries an increased risk of postoperative morbidity). There are two types of allografts depending on the treatment applied to the harvested bone: lyophilized allograft called Freeze-Dried Bone Allograft (FDBA) and demineralized lyophilized allograft called Demineralized Freeze-Dried Bone Allograft (DFDBA) or Demineralized Bone Matrix (DBM). To obtain FDBA, the harvested bone undergoes a series of treatments [11]: elimination of residual muscular and fibrous tissues, size reduction to obtain particles of 5 mm, first decontamination, microbial treatment with antibacterial, antifungal and antimycotic solutions, freezing in liquid nitrogen at −80°C, dehydration by lyophilization, second size reduction of particles, packaging in a sterile container, and finally sterilization with gamma rays to reduce the risk of contamination. FDBA will mainly serve as a matrix for bone regeneration: osteoconduction.

For the DFDBA, the treatment sequence is similar but with an additional demineralization phase in a bath of hydrochloric acid following the second reduction in particle size. The DFDBA has osteoconductive properties, meaning it serves as a scaffold for the colonization of the recipient site by various types of cells and growth factors, and some authors have shown that it has osteoinductive properties, meaning it may allow for new bone formation. This is due to the presence of Bone Morphogenetic Proteins (BMPs) within the bone matrix [12, 13]. As the bone is resorbed, growth factors including BMPs, which belong to the TGF β superfamily and were first isolated in the 1960s by American orthopedic surgeon Marshal Urist, are released. BMPs, especially isoforms 2, 3, 4, and 7, play a crucial role in bone healing by stimulating the differentiation of mesenchymal stem cells into bone cells [13].

The ability of DFDBA to be osteoconductive and osteoinductive is influenced by various factors such as the age of the donor (better between 41 and 50 years for men and 51 and 60 years for women), the particle size which should be between 500 and 710 μm to ensure optimal effects, the residual calcium content (optimal osteoinduction occurs when the percentage of residual calcium is 2%) [14], as well as the methods of preparation, sterilization, and preservation [15]. It has been shown that there is a large variation in the amounts of extracted proteins within different lots of DFDBA, and the authors have hypothesized that some proteins may be degraded within certain lots of DFDBA or present in too small quantities within the bone matrix to be detectable by their method [13].

2.1.3 Autologous platelet concentrates as surgical adjuvants

The use of autologous platelet concentrates (PRP and PRF) in oral and implant surgery aims to accelerate and improve the healing process, particularly in surgical procedures for bone regeneration [16]. Platelet Rich Plasma (PRP), introduced by Marx et al. in 1998, is obtained through two successive centrifugations in tubes containing citrate dextrose A anticoagulant (to prevent platelet activation and degranulation). The platelet concentrate is instantaneously gelled by the addition of bovine thrombin, recombinant human thrombin, or recombinant human tissue factor, which triggers platelet activation and fibrin polymerization [17].

Authors have developed a simplified protocol to obtain an autologous platelet concentrate without the use of anticoagulants or thrombin, called Platelet-Rich-Fibrin (PRF) [18]. Venous blood collected without anticoagulant is immediately centrifuged for 10 to 12 minutes at 2700–3000 rpm. The authors obtain three successive layers from the bottom to the surface of the tube: red blood cells, a PRF clot rich in platelets, and on the surface, acellular plasma rich in fibrin (**Figure 3**).

The natural mechanism of coagulation is triggered when blood comes into contact with the glass tube surface, leading to the formation of a fibrin clot rich in platelets and white blood cells without any biochemical modifications, without the addition of anticoagulant, thrombin, or calcium chloride. PRF can be used in the form of a gel or membrane.

After centrifugation, the portion rich in platelets can be mixed with the biomaterial (**Figure 4**), while the portion rich in fibrin can be transformed into a membrane by applying pressure between two compresses (**Figure 5**).

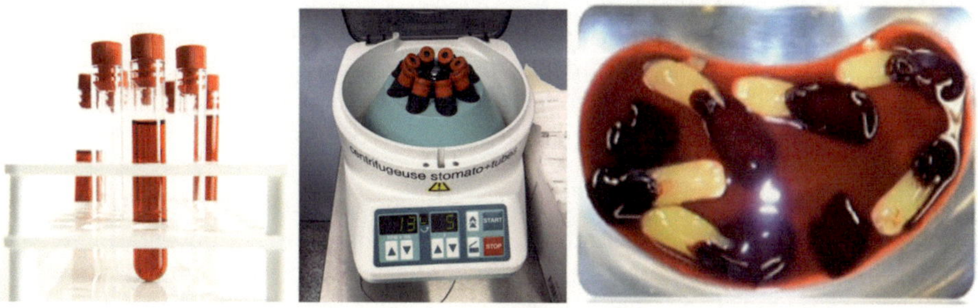

Figure 3.
Blood tubes collected from the patient without the addition of anticoagulant are placed in a centrifuge and spun at 3000 rpm for 10 minutes. This results in a material consisting of a portion rich in fibrin (in yellow), a portion rich in erythrocytes (in red), and a PRF clot rich in platelets located between them.

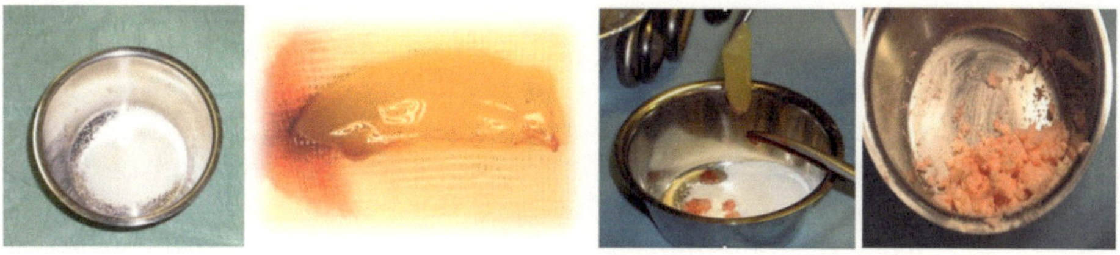

Figure 4.
300–500 μm particulate demineralized bone matrix (DFDBA). The platelet-rich portion is located at the boundary between the fibrin-rich and red blood cell-rich portions. It can be cut and mixed with DFDBA.

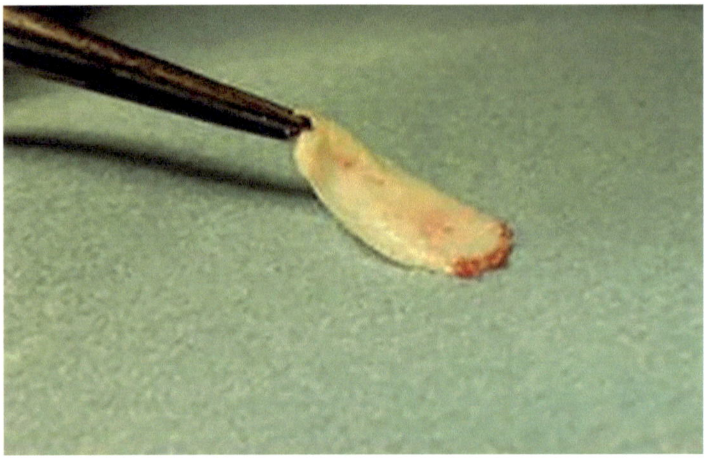

Figure 5.
The fibrin-rich portion can be manually pressed between two compresses to obtain autologous fibrin membranes.

PRF has the advantage over PRP of being entirely autologous, and it has been shown to release platelet growth factors over a period of at least 1 week [19], unlike PRP, which releases them within an hour of preparation [20]. Due to its ease of obtention, purely autologous nature, and the fact that the coagulation cascade occurs physiologically without the addition of bovine thrombin, PRF tends to replace PRP currently.

Platelet concentrates contain fibrinogen, cell adhesion molecules (fibrin, fibronectin, and vitronectin) that play a role in cell migration and osteoconduction, as well as growth factors such as PDGF (Platelet-Derived Growth Factor), TGF-β, EGF (Epithelial Growth Factor), IGF (Insulin-like Growth Factor), and VEGF (Vascular Endothelial Growth Factor) [19]. In oral implant surgery, platelet concentrates are used as adjuvants to bone reconstruction procedures. The aim of their use is to accelerate and improve the healing process, particularly in terms of bone graft integration and regeneration [21].

They are used in various clinical applications, such as maxillary sinus augmentation, alveolar ridge augmentation, mandibular reconstruction, treatment of periodontal pockets, post-extraction alveolar bone filling, and dental implant osseointegration [22–25]. Studies have shown the beneficial effects of platelet concentrates, such as improved soft tissue healing [26, 27]. However, the improvement of bone regeneration through platelet concentrate administration is still controversial [28, 29]. The lack of standardization in platelet concentrate obtention protocols may explain the lack of concordance in various studies, and the kinetics of growth factor delivery is still poorly understood, with large variations observed among patients and even within the same patient depending on the time of day of the blood collection (circadian variations in platelet concentration exist) [18, 19]. Furthermore, the contradictory results reported in the literature regarding the benefits of using platelet coagulation factors can be partly explained by the fact that these results come from clinical studies for some and animal studies for others, and it is difficult to extrapolate results obtained from one species to another [30, 31].

On the other hand, the minimum platelet concentration required to obtain a blood clot meeting the criteria for PRF is not well defined by the authors. However, they agree that clinical benefits can be obtained for a platelet concentration of 1 million/μL of plasma (4 to 7 times the baseline level) [32].

2.1.4 Use of a combination of allograft and platelet concentrates

The benefits associated with the use of a combination of biomaterials, such as allograft and platelet concentrates, are currently still controversial. One study [33] compared the use of a bone allograft alone with a bone allograft combined with platelet-rich fibrin (PRF) for maxillary sinus augmentation in 9 patients. According to the authors, the combination of allograft and PRF allows for faster bone maturity, which enables dental implant placement at 4 months postoperatively compared to 8 months for the control group.

The clinical benefits of platelet concentrates combined with demineralized freeze-dried bone allograft (DFDBA) in bone regeneration have been demonstrated in the treatment of periodontal pockets [34, 35], but have not yet been evaluated in oral surgery in a large cohort of patients.

2.2 Surgical techniques

2.2.1 Principles of post-extraction alveolar ridge preservation

Post-extraction alveolar ridge preservation techniques are based on the principle of guided bone regeneration. The principle involves placing a membrane between the soft tissues and the alveolar bone contours. This membrane prevents the passage and proliferation of epithelial cells and connective tissue into the alveolus, thus ensuring a space that can be colonized by osteoprogenitor cells. This prevents the growth and invagination of soft tissues into the extraction site during healing, thus allowing for adequate bone preservation. In addition to its role in maintaining space, the membrane stabilizes, protects, and ensures the containment of the blood clot and, optionally, the graft material that has been inserted into the alveolus. The biomaterial placed in the dental alveolus under the membrane immediately after extraction will constitute a structure whose architecture will guide and support colonization by osteoprogenitor cells and, thereby, bone regeneration. The Alveolar Ridge preservation Technique Using DFDBA and Platelet Concentrates The Implantology Clinic at Erasme Hospital routinely uses a combination of DFDBA bone bank and PRF platelet concentrates in the form of gel and membrane during post-extraction alveolar ridge preservation procedures. At the start of surgery, 6 to 8 tubes of 10 ml blood without anticoagulants are collected from the patient. Centrifugation at 3000 rpm for 10 minutes or 2800 rpm for 12 minutes is performed according to a protocol described in a previous study [18]. The platelet-rich portion (which is at the boundary between the yellow fibrin-rich part and the red erythrocyte-rich part) is collected and mixed with particulate allograft (DFDBA) with a particle size of 300 to 500 μm. The fibrin-rich portion is manually pressed between two compresses to obtain autologous fibrin membranes. Atraumatic extractions are performed, and immediately thereafter, the alveolar ridge is filled with the DFDBA-platelet concentrate mixture. Closure of the alveolus is ensured by the fibrin membrane, and resorbable sutures (Vicryl® 3/0) are performed (**Figure 6**).

Immediately after atraumatic extraction, the alveolar ridge is augmented using a mixture of DFDBA and platelet concentrates. The alveolar ridge is closed using a fibrin membrane and absorbable sutures (Vicryl® 3/0). During the post-operative period, 600 mg of ibuprofen three times a day and 500 mg of paracetamol are prescribed for pain relief. All patients receive 1 g of amoxicillin twice a day for 4 days or 300 mg of clindamycin three times a day if allergic to penicillin, for 4 days. This technique provides good results in terms of preserving post-extractional bone volume [36].

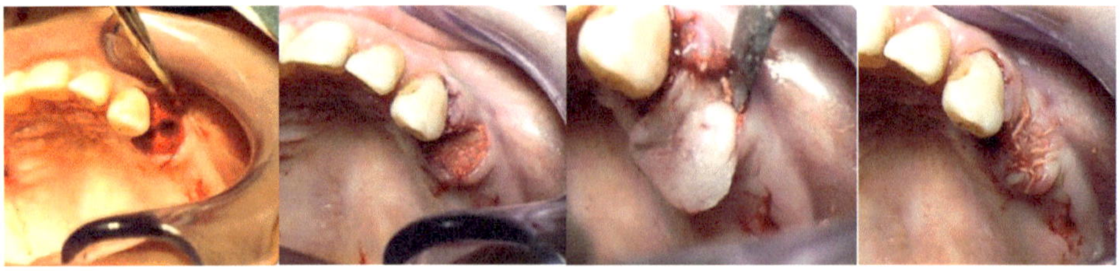

Figure 6.
Post-extractional alveolar ridge augmentation technique as practiced in the Implantology Clinic of Erasme Hospital.

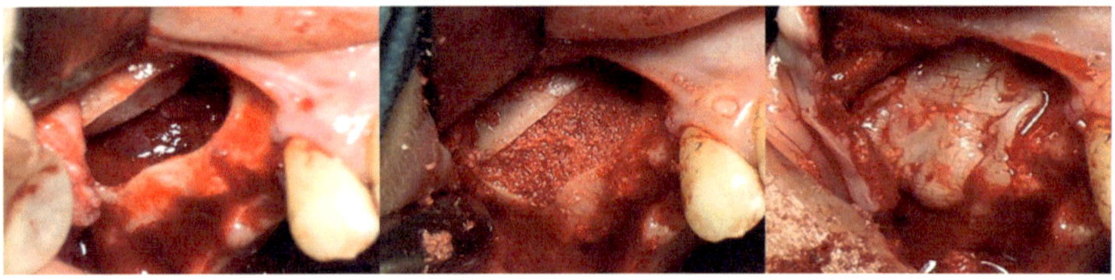

Figure 7.
Procedure for maxillary sinus grafting as performed at the implantology clinic of Erasme Hospital. A bone flap is made with piezoelectric surgery on the antero-external wall of the right maxillary sinus, followed by horizontal tipping while lifting the Schneider membrane of the sinus. Autologous fibrin membranes are placed on the internal, anterior, and posterior walls of the cavity, and then a mixture of DFDBA and autologous platelet concentrates is placed in the cavity. Autologous fibrin membranes are then applied outside the graft, and the mucoperiosteal flap is sutured in place.

2.2.2 Sinus lift

There are different techniques for augmenting the maxillary sinus floor to create adequate bone volume. Studies have shown that the results of maxillary sinus grafting in terms of implant survival rates are best when using only biomaterial as the grafting material, with 96.0% implant survival rate at 5 years when using 100% biomaterial versus 87.8% when using autogenous bone [36].

The technique we use in the Implantology Clinic of Erasme Hospital is based on the insertion of a mixture consisting exclusively of DFDBA and platelet concentrates under the Schneiderian membrane of the maxillary sinus, after creating a bone flap using piezo surgery at the antero-external wall of the maxillary sinus. Autologous fibrin membranes are placed on the walls of the cavity, followed by a mixture of DFDBA and autologous platelet concentrates, which is obtained as described in the previous chapter. Autologous fibrin membranes are then applied outside the graft, and the mucoperiosteal flap is sutured in place (**Figure 7**).

3. Bone quality

It has become crucial in contemporary implantology to keep the alveolar ridge after extraction. There is currently agreement that alveolar ridge maintenance is necessary to prevent further bone loss [36, 37]. According to a recent study, the combination of PRF platelet concentrates with particle DFDBA (300–500 m) results in excellent outcomes for post-extractional bone preservation [36].

Alveolar ridge preservation and sinus lift procedures enable the favorable conservation or restoration of bone volume; however, for medium- and long-term implant results, it is also crucial to objectively evaluate the quality of the acquired reconstruction. To achieve this, authors frequently employ histomorphometry, a method for examining both qualitative and quantitative aspects of bone quality [37–40].

A. Wardani et al.'s recent work used DFDBA (300–500) and PRF platelet concentrate to assess bone quality in sinus lift and alveolar socket preservation. 40 2 mm-diameter bone samples from 21 patients were the subject of an interventional prospective investigation. In order to serve as control groups, 22 biopsies were taken from preserved sockets, 7 from grafted sinus locations, and 11 from native bone [37].

The samples were fixed, embedded in paraffin, sliced on a microtome, and then stained with Masson's trichrome and hematoxylin-eosin.

According to the ratios of woven (immature) and lamellar (mature) bone, a healing score ranging from 1 to 3 was given to each bone sample to make it easier to compare them. Score 1 showed a predominance of woven bone (difference between woven and lamellar bone proportion > 10%) and reflected an early stage of bone healing; score 2 showed the presence of lamellar and woven bone in similar proportions (difference between woven and lamellar bone proportion 10%) and reflected a moderate stage of bone healing; and score 3 showed a predominance of lamellar bone (difference between woven and lam) (**Table 1**).

3.1 Native bone samples

The majority of the native bone samples displayed a score of 3 (9/11), which denotes extensive bone repair. Only two samples (**Table 2**) got a score of 2, corresponding to a moderate level of healing. Only lamellar bone was visible in two samples, which indicates extraordinarily high bone density. Remember that the mandibular symphysis bone is where these samples originated. Lamellar bone made up an average of 52.73% of native bone, woven bone made up an average of 10.74% of native bone, and overall bone made up an average of 65.29% of native bone. Native bone received an average healing score of 2.82.

3.2 Alveolar samples

Table 3 contains a list of the samples collected from grafted alveolar structures. A score of 1 was assigned to two out of the 22 samples, which were eliminated after 3 and 5 months of healing, respectively. Except for four samples that were obtained after 5 months had passed since the start of the healing process, 12 out of 22 samples

Bone healing score	
1	Prevalence of woven bone (difference in the proportions of woven and lamellar bone >10%)
2	Lamellar and woven bon in similar proportions (difference in the proportions of woven and lamellar bone <10%)
3	Prevalence of lamellar bone (difference in the proportions of woven and lamellar bone >10%)

Table 1.
Bone healing score.

Native bone sample	Proportion of total bone (%)	Proportion of lamellar bone (%)	Proportion of woven bone	Score
Sample 1	44.31	44.15	0.15%	3
Sample 2	39.45	39.45	0.00%	3
Sample 3	48.13	45.45	2.67%	3
Sample 4	44.69	42.80	1.89%	3
Sample 5	48.64	46.23	2.40%	3
Sample 6	91.01	91.01	0	3
Sample 7	83.54	83.54	0	3
Sample 8	85.40	42.50	42.90%	2
Sample 9	65.60	39.10	26.50%	3
Sample 10	70.10	61.20	8.90%	3
Sample 11	97.4	44.70	52.70%	2
Mean	65.29	52.73	10.74%	2.82

Table 2.
Proportion of bone surfaces in native bone.

(**Figures 8–11**) had a score of 2. **Table 3** shows that 8 out of 22 samples received a 3 rating. Alveolar structure samples were divided into two groups based on whether the healing duration was less than (A) or higher than (B) 5 months. In comparison to group A, the samples in group B had a higher average proportion of newly produced bone and a lower average proportion of DFDBA residual particles (**Table 4**).

3.3 Sinus lift samples

Table 5 displays the samples taken from sinus lifts. The samples, all except one of which had a score of 3, were collected between six and 9 months after healing (**Figures 12** and **13**). A single sample was taken 8 months into the healing process and had a score of 2 (**Table 5**).

According to the study, as healing time increases, there is a greater proportion of lamellar neoformed bone than unformed tissue (**Figure 8**). The amount of newly produced bone in the grafted sockets significantly increased as healing progressed (average: 41.22% 5 months, 55.89% > 5 months). Additionally, it appears that DFDBA particle resorption and healing time in the grafted socket are associated (average: 15.43 5 months, 13.72% > 5 months). When utilizing DFDBA and PRF for sinus lift and alveolar socket preservation, high-quality, mature bone tissue is produced that meets histological standards [37].

In the present investigation, samples taken from native bone were examined, and it was shown that 10.72% of the samples (8 out of 11) included immature woven bone, which is probably the result of normal bone remodeling [41, 42]. Furthermore, lamellar bone was only present in two native bone samples, making up more than 80% of the sample area and indicating advanced bone maturity. With an average healing score of 2.32 and a majority of lamellar bone, all 22 samples tested from grafted alveoli showed freshly created bone. The average percentage of newly produced bone across all prepared cell samples was 46.56%, demonstrating the effectiveness of

Samples	Δt (healing time prior to sampling in months)	Proportion of newly formed bone (%)	Proportion of residual DFDBA particles (%)	Score
Sample 1	2	38.76	16.10	2
Sample 2	3	21.89	7.10	1
Sample 3	3	52.80	20.10	2
Sample 4	3	83.10	14.20	3
Sample 5	4	45.10	29.60	3
Sample 6	4	76.60	20.20	3
Sample 7	4	38.60	32.30	2
Sample 8	4.5	45.20	31.10	2
Sample 9	5	5.15	18.91	1
Sample 10	5	22.04	12.31	2
Sample 11	5	30.64	4.22	2
Sample 12	5	25.90	3 .45	2
Sample 13	5	75.99	0.91	3
Sample 14	5	15.44	5.54	2
Sample 15	6	69.60	12.70	2
Sample 16	7	45.70	2.33	3
Sample 17	7.5	72.90	17.50	2
Sample 18	7.5	54.70	37.40	2
Sample 19	9	36.55	5.90	3
Sample 20	9	31.32	8.59	3
Sample 21	15	63.40	5.40	2
Sample 22	15	73.00	20.00	3
Mean	—	46.29	14.81	2.27

Table 3.
Proportions of newly formed bone surface, residual particles, and healing score of samples from alveolar grafted sockets.

using PRF and DFDBA alveolar fillers to encourage bone neoformation. The average percentage of newly produced bone in samples collected within the first 5 months of recovery was 41.22%, but the average percentage in samples taken more than 5 months later was 55.89%.

An average proportion of newly produced bone of 47.41% was seen 4 months after healing in a previous histomorphometric study that used DFDBA without PRF [42], which is marginally greater than the proportion attained in the current study. It was noticed that the DFDBA (donor variability) origin difference in our study may have had an impact on the outcomes.

Our study found an average of 15.43% at healing periods less than or equal to 5 months and an average of 13.72% at healing periods more than 5 months, indicating gradual resorption of the allograft particles over time. This proportion of residual DFDBA particles was found to exist within the grafted alveoli. According to a recent study [43], there were 37.42% residual DFDBA particles at 2 months and

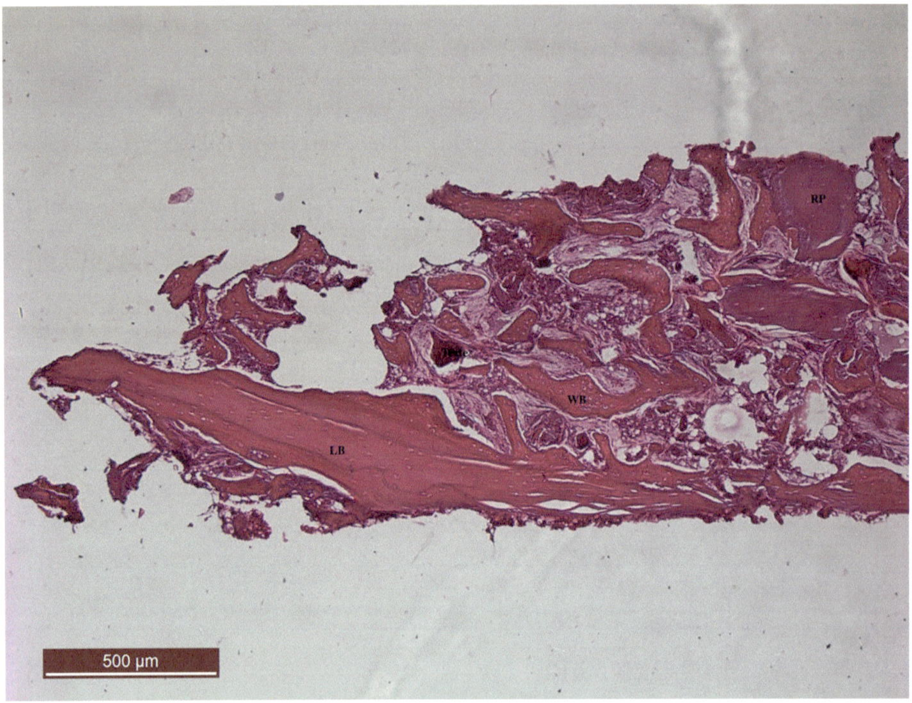

Figure 8.
Sample from a grafted alveolar socket showing a healing score of 2 (H&E). Lamellar bone (LB), woven bone (WB), residual particle (RP).

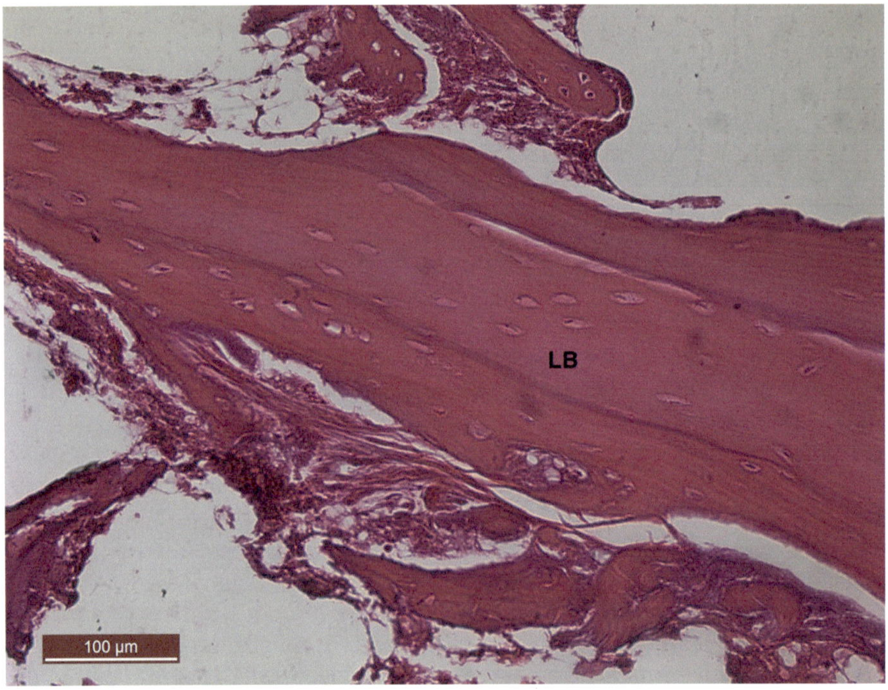

Figure 9.
Sample from a grafted alveolar socket showing a healing score of 2 (H&E). Lamellar bone (LB).

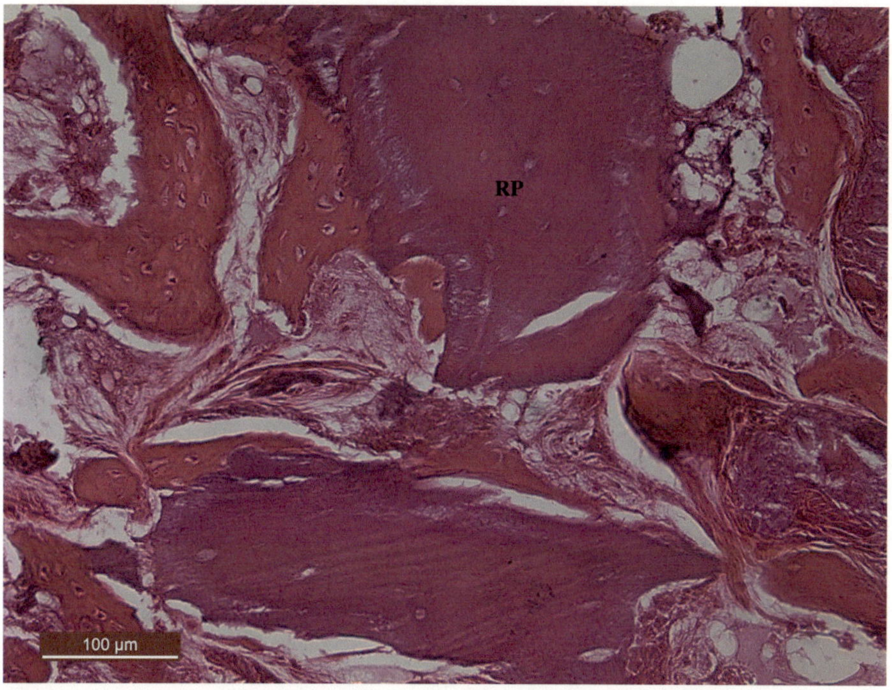

Figure 10.
Sample from a grafted alveolar socket showing a healing score of 2 (H&E). Residual particle (RP).

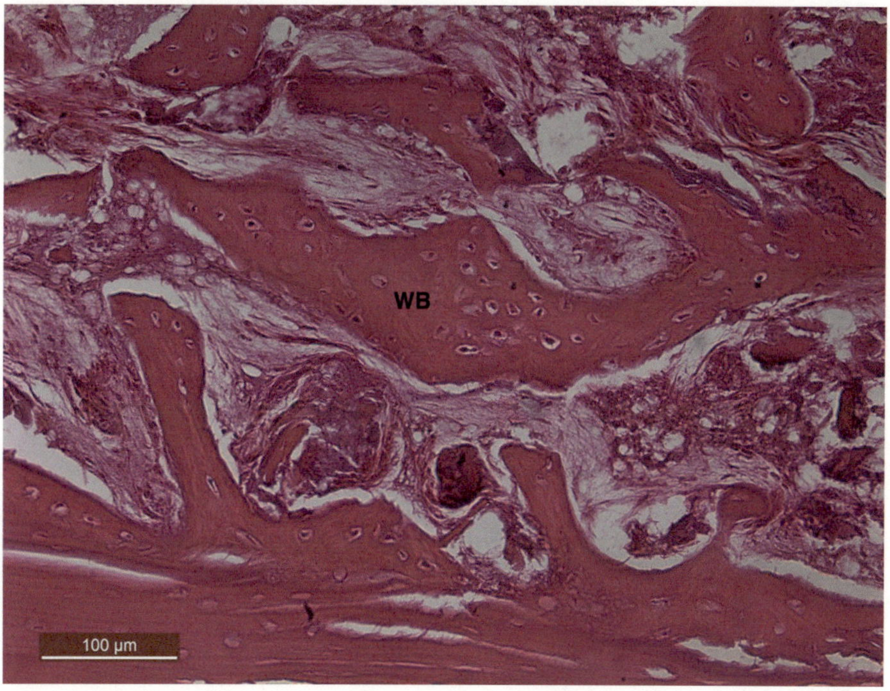

Figure 11.
Sample from a grafted alveolar socket showing a healing score of 2 (H&E). Woven bone (WB).

	Average proportion of newly formed bone (%)	Average proportion of residual particle (%)	Average healing score
≤5 months	41.42	15.43	2.14
>5 months	55.89	13.72	2.5

Table 4.
Average proportions as a function of the healing time for alveolar grafted sockets.

Bone samples in sinus lifts	Δt(healing time prior to sampling in months)	Proportion of newly formed bone (%)	Proportion of residual DFDBA particles (%)	Healing score
Sample 1	6	82.90	9.60	3
Sample 2	6	41.40	24.60	3
Sample 3	7	26.88	13.72	3
Sample 4	7.5	36.88	6.47	3
Sample 5	8	63.50	13.90	3
Sample 6	8	48.20	20.10	2
Sample 7	9	40.24	3.09	3
Mean	—	48.57	13.07	2.86

Table 5.
Proportions of newly formed bone, residual particles, and healing score of sinus lifts.

26.80% at 4 months. This suggests that particles in our study were absorbed more quickly.

The study found a propensity to see equal amounts of both at healing durations of less than 5 months with regard to the proportions of lamellar and woven bone, indicative of bone maturity. In contrast, there was a tendency toward a predominance of lamellar bone after 5 months of healing, which suggests that the graft evolved over time toward better bone maturity. These results suggest that the post-extraction alveolar arrangement using particle DFDBA (300–500 m) and A-PRF produces good results in terms of bone quality and maturity. It is difficult to compare these findings with other histomorphometric studies because many of them just look at the overall proportion of freshly created bone rather than distinguishing between lamellar and woven bone.

After 6 to 9 months, samples from the locations that received a sinus lift revealed an average proportion of newly produced bone of 48.57% in all seven samples, with a higher proportion of lamellar bone (scoring 3) than woven bone in six of the seven samples. This demonstrates that sinus grafts that were treated with particulate DFDBA (300–500 m) and PRF successfully healed the bone.

In a different study [43], sinus lift patients were divided into two groups: one with DFDBA alone and the other with DFDBA with PRF. At 6 months, the group with PRF had a larger percentage of newly created bone (18.35%) than the group without PRF (12.95%), indicating that PRF has a beneficial effect on new bone production.

As comparing these findings to those of our study, it appears that DFDBA and PRF for sinus lift produce superior results in terms of new bone creation as compared

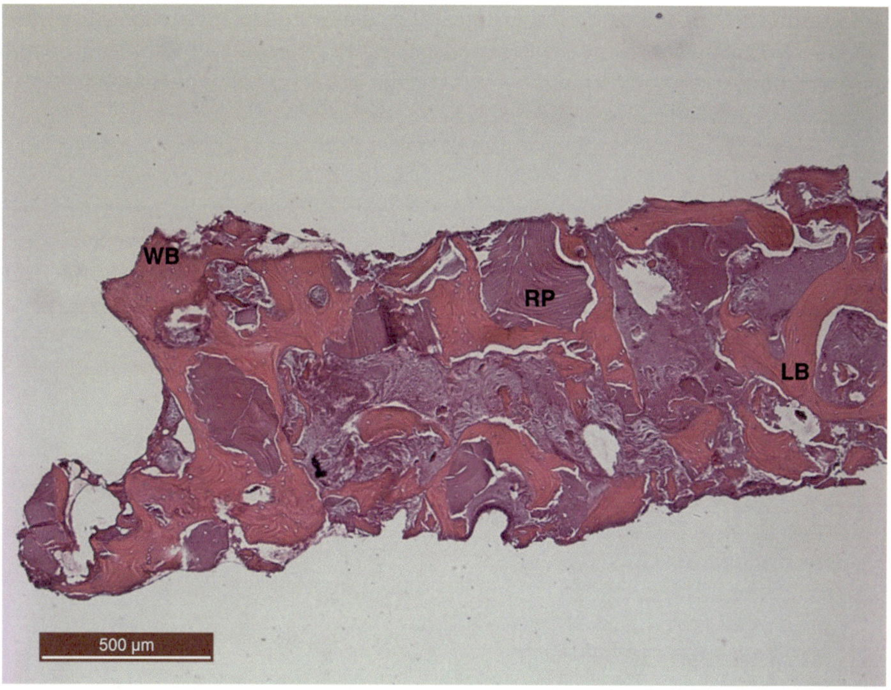

Figure 12.
Sample from a sinus lift displaying a healing score of 3 (H&E). Woven bone (WB), lamellar bone (LB), residual particle (RP).

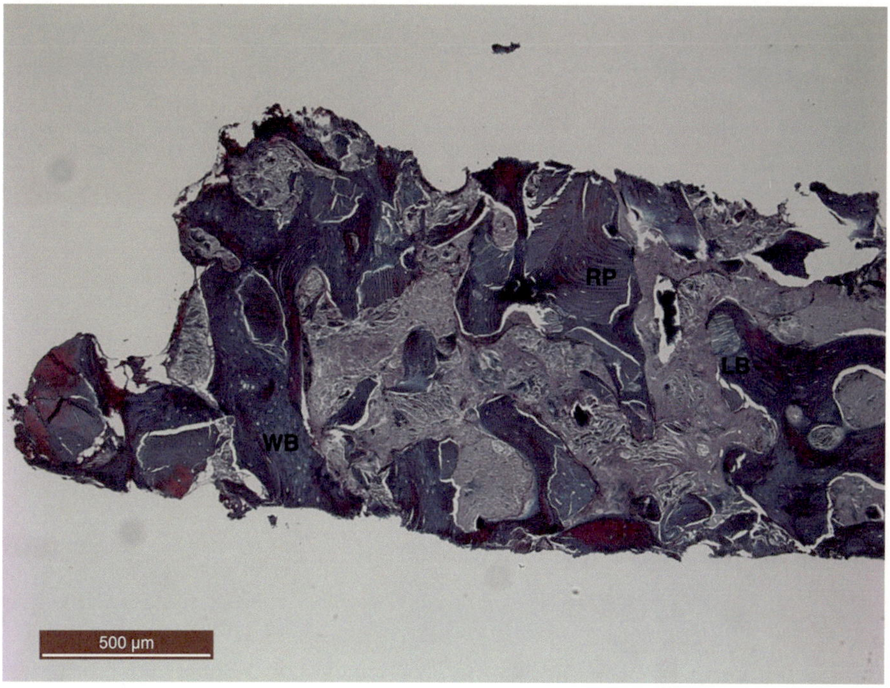

Figure 13.
Sample from a sinus lift displaying a healing score of 3 (TM). Woven bone (WB), lamellar bone (LB), residual particle (RP).

to DBBM and PRF. By exposing lingering BMPs, the osteoinductive capability of DFDBA—a product of its demineralization during preparation—might be able to explain this discrepancy. However, because of the small sample size in our study, additional research with bigger sample sizes is preferred to improve the findings. We found 13.07% of residual particles in the sinus lift samples, with an average healing time of 7.35 months.

After an average healing duration of 10.81 months, histomorphometric analysis of samples taken without sinus lifts using FDBA and DFDBA revealed an average proportion of residual particles of 9.56% and 10.11%, respectively [44]. These findings are consistent with our research and point to a long-term beneficial absorption of allograft particles after sinus lift surgeries.

4. Conclusion

For post-extractional alveolar ridge augmentation and sinus lift surgeries, the combination of 300–500 m DFDBA and autologous platelet-rich concentrate, such as PRF, yields predictable clinical results.

Conflict of interest

The authors declare no conflict of interest.

Author details

Adnane Wardani[1*] and Laurence Evrard[2]

1 Dentistry Department, Hôpital Universitaire de Bruxelles (HUB), Belgium

2 Oral and Maxillofacial Surgery Department, Hôpital Universitaire de Bruxelles (HUB), Université Libre de Bruxelles, Erasme Site, Belgium

*Address all correspondence to: adnanewardani@gmail.com

References

[1] Araújo MG, Lindhe J, et al. Socket grafting with the use of autologous bone: An experimental study in the dog. Clinical Oral Implants Research. 2011;**22**(1):9-13

[2] Van der Weijden F, Dell'Acqua F, et al. Alveolar bone dimensional changes of post-extraction sockets in humans: A systematic review. Journal of Clinical Periodontology. 2009;**36**(12):1048-1058

[3] Covani U, Ricci M, Bozzolo G, Mangano F, Zini A, Barone A. Analysis of the pattern of the alveolar ridge remodeling following single tooth extraction. Clinical Oral Implants Research. 2011;**22**(8):820-825

[4] Oikarinen K, Raustia AM, Hartikainen M. General and local contraindications for endosseal implants--an epidemiological panoramic radiograph study in 65-year-old subjects. Community Dentistry and Oral Epidemiology. 1995;**23**(2):114-118

[5] Vignoletti F, Matesanz P, et al. Surgical protocols for ridge preservation after tooth extraction a systematic review. Clinical Oral Implants Research. 2012;**23**(Suppl. 5):22-38

[6] Ten Heggeler JM, Slot DE, et al. Effect of socket preservation therapies following tooth extraction in non-molar regions in humans: A systematic review. Clinical Oral Implants Research. 2011;**22**(8):779-788

[7] Van den Bergh JPA, ten Bruggenkate CM, Krekeler G, Tuinzing DB. Maxillary sinus floor elevation and grafting with human demineralized freeze dried bone. Clinical Oral Implantaion Research. 2000;**11**:487-493

[8] Mazor Z, Peleg M, Gross M. Sinus augmentation for single tooth replacement in the posterior maxilla: A 3-year follow-up. The International Journal of Oral & Maxillofacial Implants. 1999;**14**:55-60

[9] Bader H et al. Immediate extraction site grafting: materials and clinical objectives. Dentistry Today. 2005;**24**(7):86-89

[10] Tischler M, Misch CE, et al. Extraction site bone grafting in general dentistry. Review of applications and principles. Dentistry Today. 2004;**23**(5):108-113

[11] Holtzclaw D, Toscano N, Eisenlohr L, Callan D. The safety of bone allografts used in dentistry: A review. Journal of American Dental Association. 2008;**139**(9):1192-1199

[12] Zhang M, Powers RM, Wolfinbarger L Jr. Effects of the demineralization process on the osteoinductivity of demineralized bone matrix. Journal of Periodontology. 1997;**68**:1085-1092

[13] Li H, Pujic Z, Xiao Y, Bartold PM. Identification of bone morphogenetic proteins 2 and 4 in commercial De mineralized freeze-dried bone allograft preparations: Pilot study. Clinical Implantation Research and Dental Related Research. 2000;**2**(2):110-117

[14] Ghanbari H, Moeintaghavi A, Sargolzaei N, Foroozanfar A, Dadpour Y. Comparativestudyofalgiporeanddecalcified freeze-dried bone allograft in open maxillary sinus elevation using piezoelectric surgery. Journal of Periodontology and Implant Dentistry. 2013;**5**(1):1-6

[15] Schwartz Z, Mellonig JT, Carnes DL, de la Fontaine J, Cochran DL, Dean BB, et al. Ability of commercial demineralized freeze-dried bone allografts. Journal of Periodontology. 1996;**67**:918-926

[16] Bayens M, Glineur R, Evrard L. L'intérêt de l'utilisation des facteurs plaquettaires de la coagulation : Platelet-Rich Plasma (PRP) et Platelet-Rich Fibrin (PRF) dans la reconstruction osseuse pré-implantaire. Revue Médicale de Bruxelles. 2010;**31**:521-527

[17] Marx RE, Carlson ER, Eichstaedt RM, Schimmele SR, Strauss JE, Georgeff KR. Platelet-rich plasma: Growth factor enhancement for bone grafts. Oral Surgery, Oral Medicine, Oral Pathology, Oral Radiology, and Endodontics. 1998;**85**:638-646

[18] Dohan DM, Choukroun J, Diss A, Dohan SL, Dohan AJ, Mouhyi J, et al. Platelet-rich fibrin (PRF): A second-generation platelet concentrate. Part I: Technological concepts and evolution. Oral Surgery, Oral Medicine, Oral Pathology, Oral Radiology, and Endodontics. 2006;**101**:37-44

[19] Dohan DM, Choukroun J, Diss A, Dohan SL, Dohan AJ, Mouhyi J, et al. Platelet-rich fibrin (PRF): A second-generation platelet concentrate. Part II: Platelet-related biologic features. Oral Surgery, Oral Medicine, Oral Pathology, Oral Radiology, and Endodontics. 2006;**101**:45-50

[20] Hallman M, Thor A. Bone substitutes and growth factors as an alternative/complement to autogenous bone for grafting in implant dentistry. Periodontology. 2000;**47**:172-192

[21] Marx RE, Garg AK. Dental and Craniofacial Applications of Platelet-Rich Plasma. UK: Quintessence Publishing Co, Inc; 2005

[22] Steigmann M, Garg AK. A comparative study of bilateral sinus lifts performed with platelet-rich plasma alone versus alloplastic graft material reconstituted with blood. Implant Dentistry. 2005;**14**:261-266

[23] Ito K, Yamada Y, Naiki T, Ueda M. Simultaneous implant placement and bone regeneration around dental implants using tissue-engineered bone with fibrin glue, mesenchymal stem cells and platelet-rich plasma. Clinical Oral Implants Research. 2006;**17**:579-586

[24] Hanna R, Trejo PM, Weltman RL. Treatment of intrabony defects with bovine-derived xenograft alone and in combination with platelet-rich plasma: A randomized clinical trial. Journal of Periodontology. 2004;**75**:1668-1677

[25] Anitua E, Orive G, Aguirre JJ, Andía I. Clinical outcome of immediately loaded dental implants bioactivated with plasma rich in growth factors: A 5-year retrospective study. Journal of Periodontology. 2008;**79**:1168-1176

[26] Choukroun J, Diss A, et al. Platelet-rich fibrin (PRF): A second-generation platelet concentrate Part IV: Clinical effects on tissue healing. Oral Surgery, Oral Medicine, Oral Pathology, Oral Radiology, and Endodontics. 2006;**101**(3):e56-e60

[27] Hom DB, Linzie BM, Huang TC. The healing effects of autologous platelet gel on acute human skin wounds. Archives of Facial Plastic Surgery. 2007;**9**(3):174-183

[28] Piemontese M, Aspriello SD, Rubini C, Ferrante L, Procaccini M. Treatment of periodontal intrabonydefects with demineralized freeze-dried bone allograft in combination with platelet-rich plasma: A comparative clinical trial. Journal of Periodontology. 2008;**79**(5):802-810

[29] Singh A, Kohli M, Gupta N. Platelet rich fibrin: A novel approach for osseous regeneration. Journal of Maxillofacial and Oral Surgery. 2012;**11**(4):430-434

[30] Casati MZ, de Vasconcelos Gurgel BC, Gonçalves PF, Pimentel SP, da Rocha Nogueira Filho G, Nociti FH, et al. Platelet-rich plasma does not improve bone regeneration around peri-implant bone defects – A pilot study in dogs. International Journal of Oral and Maxillofacial Surgery. 2007;**36**:132-136

[31] Gürbüzer B, Pikdöken L, Urhan M, Süer BT, Narin Y. Scintigraphic evaluation of early osteoblastic activity in extraction sockets treated with platelet-rich plasma. Journal of Oral and Maxillofacial Surgery. 2008;**66**:2454-2460

[32] Weibrich G, Hansen T, Kleis W, Buch R, Hitzler WE. Effect of platelet concentration in platelet-rich plasma on peri-implant bone regeneration. Bone. 2004;**34**:665-671

[33] Choukroun J, Diss A, Simonpieri A, Girard MO, Schoeffler C, Dohan SL, et al. Platelet-rich fibrin (PRF): A second-generation plateletconcentrate. Part V: Histologic evaluations of PRF effects on bone allograft maturation in sinus lift. Oral Surgery, Oral Medicine, Oral Pathology, Oral Radiology, and Endodontics. 2006;**101**:299-303

[34] Bansal C, Bharti V. Evaluation of efficacy of autologous platelet-rich fibrin with demineralized-freeze dried bone allograft in the treatment of periodontal intrabony defects. Journal of Indian Society of Periodontology. 2013;**17**(3):361-366

[35] Markou N, Pepelassi E, Kotsovilis S, et al. The use of platelet-rich plasma combined with demineralized freeze-dried bone allograft in the treatment of periodontal endosseous defects: A report of two clinical cases. Journal of the American Dental Association (1939). 2010;**141**(8):967-978

[36] Baniasadi B, Evrard L. Alveolar ridge preservation after tooth extraction with DFDBA and platelet concentrates: A radiographic retrospective study. The Open Dentistry Journal. 2017;**14**:99-108

[37] Wardani A, et al. Healing of particulate allografts mixed with platelet concentrates in ridge preservation and sinus lift: A prospective histomorphometric study. Morphologie. Sep 2023;**107**(358):100596

[38] Geurs N, Ntounis A, Vassilopoulos P, Vandervelden U, Loos B, Reddy M. Using growth factors in human extraction sockets: A histologic and histomorphometric evaluation of short-term healing. International Journal of Oral and Maxillofacial Implants. 2014;**29**:485-496

[39] Zhan Y, Stefan G, Tangl C, Huber D, Lixin Qiu Y. PRF effects of Choukroun's platelet-rich fibrin on bone regeneration in combination with deproteinized bovine bone mineral in maxillary sinus augmentation: A histological and histomorphometric study. Journal of Cranio Maxillofacial Surgery. 2012;**40**:321-328

[40] Hatakeyama M, Beletti E, Zanetta-Barbosa D, Dechichi P. Radiographic and histomorphometric analysis of bone healing using autogenous graft associated with platelet-rich plasma obtained by 2 different methods. Oral Surgery, Oral Medicine, Oral Pathology, Oral Radiology, and Endodontics. 2008;**105**:8-13

[41] Desoutter J, Mentaverri R, Brazier M, Kamel S. Physiological and pathological

bone remodeling. Revue Francophone des laboratoires. 2012;**446**:33-42

[42] Whetman J, Mealey B. Effect of healing time on new bone formation following tooth extraction and ridge preservation with demineralized freeze-dried bone allograft. A randomized controlled clinical trial. Journal of Periodontology. 2016;**87**:147-160

[43] Zhang Y, Tangl S, Huber CD, Lin Y, Qiu L, Rausch X. Effects of Choukroun's platelet-rich fibrin on bone regeneration in combination with deproteinized bovine bone mineral in maxillary sinus augmentation: A histological and histomorphometric study. Journal of Cranio-Maxillo-Facial Surgery. 2012;**40**:321-328

[44] Cammack GV, Nevins M, Clem DS, Hatch JP, Mellonig JT. Histologic evaluation of mineralized and demineralized freeze-dried bone allograft for ridge and sinus augmentations. The International Journal of Periodontics & Restorative Dentistry. 2005;**25**:231-237

Chapter 9

The Combined Use of Particulate Allografts (DFDBA) and Platelet Concentrates in Oral and Maxillo-Facial Surgery

Laurence Evrard

Abstract

Among the biomaterials used in the field of oral surgery, allogeneic bone is considered as a good material. In the particulate form, demineralized freeze-dried bone allograft (DFDBA) is useful in many procedures in maxillofacial surgery. Platelet concentrate (platelet-rich fibrin, PRF) is obtained by centrifugation of blood. This contains high concentrations of growth factors and could enhance healing, and possibly improve bone repair and regeneration. Although it remains unclear whether they are able to accelerate bone healing and influence bone quality, platelet concentrates accelerate dermal soft tissue and oral mucosa healing post-extraction. A combination of particulate DFDBA and platelet concentrate (PRF) is used in our department for horizontal and vertical bone grafts.

Keywords: allograft, platelet concentrate, PRF, DFDBA, bone reconstruction

1. Introduction

Autogenous bone has long been considered the gold standard for bone reconstruction in maxillo-facial surgery. However, the current trend is to increasingly use biomaterials as an alternative to autogenous bone, with the aim of reducing post-operative morbidity related to the act of bone harvesting at the donor site, and to reduce the operating time.

2. Biomaterials used in oral and maxillo-facial surgery

Biomaterials used in oral surgery are classified into two categories: biomaterials of natural origin and biomaterials of synthetic origin. For review, see [1].

2.1 Biomaterials of synthetic origin

Biomaterials of synthetic origin are tricalcium phosphate, hydroxyapatites, two-phase ceramics, bioactive glasses, and polymers.

Tricalcium phosphates (ßTCP) $Ca_3(PO_4)_2$ are produced by heating a mixture of calcium phosphate powder and naphthalene to over a thousand degrees and under pressure, which, after sublimation, leaves a porous structure that gives rise to the osteoconductive properties of the material.

The porous hydroxyapatite $Ca_{10}(PO_4)_6(OH)_2$ is obtained by the thermal transformation of calcium carbonate. Chemically, this calcium phosphate is the closest to biological apatite crystals. Several porosities are available. The higher the porosity, the better the osteoconduction.

Two-phase ceramics (biphasic calcium phosphate (BCP)) include a combination of hydroxyapatite and tricalcium phosphate in different proportions, which make it possible to combine the qualities of the two materials, in particular to obtain adequate resorption and mechanical qualities.

Bioglasses, SiO_2-P_2O_5-CaO-NaO, are materials called "bioactive". This "bioactivity" would take place due to surface reactions of the bioglass and ion exchanges with biological fluids. The bioactive bone/glass bond would take place through a layer of amorphous silica gel which would exert a chemotactic effect on the osteoblasts. Polymers with, in particular polymethylmethacrylate (PMMA), have excellent biocompatibility.

2.2 Biomaterials of natural origin

The biomaterials of natural origin are xenogenic bone, natural coral and allogeneic bone.

Xenogenic bone (xenograft) is most often of porcine or bovine origin. Inorganic bovine bone retains a bony spatial structure, giving it osteoconductive properties. These are products presented in freeze-dried form [2]. Natural coral is 99% calcium carbonate. After heat treatment, it retains a porous structure that gives it osteoinductive properties [2].

Allogeneic bone substitutes are produced from femoral head bone taken from human individuals (fresh corpse). Compared to autogenous bone, they have the advantage of not requiring harvesting from the patient (in fact, the harvesting of autogenous bone is accompanied by an increased risk of post-operative morbidity). There are two types of allograft depending on the treatment applied to the harvested bone: freeze-dried allograft called the Freeze Dried Bone Allograft (FDBA) and freeze-dried demineralized allograft called the Demineralized Freeze Dried Bone Allograft (DFDBA) or Demineralized Bone Matric (DBM).

To obtain the FDBA, the bone removed will undergo a series of treatments such as [3]: the elimination of residual musculo-fibrous tissue, size reduction until 5 mm particles are obtained, initial decontamination, microbial treatment with antibacterial, antifungal, and antiviral solutions, freezing in liquid nitrogen at −80°C, dehydration by freeze-drying, a second reduction in particle size, packaging in sterile packaging, and finally sterilization with gamma rays to reduce the risk of contamination. The FDBA will mainly serve as a matrix for bone regeneration: osteoconduction.

For DFDBA, the treatment sequence is similar but with a demineralization phase in a hydrochloric acid bath, which is added following the second reduction in particle size.

Demineralized freeze-dried bone allograft (DFDBA) has osteoconductive properties, that is, it serves as a scaffold for the colonization of the recipient site by different cell types and growth factors, and some authors have shown that it has osteoinductive properties; that is to say that it would allow the neoformation of bone. This would take place due to the presence of Bone Morphogenetic Proteins (BMPs) within the bone matrix [4, 5]. Indeed, as it resorbs, the bone releases growth factors, including BMPs belonging to the transforming growth factor beta (TGF β) superfamily and isolated for the first time in the 1960s by Marshall Urist, an American orthopedic surgeon. BMPs and, in particular, isoforms 2, 3, 4, and 7 play a crucial role in bone healing by stimulating the differentiation of mesenchymal stem cells into bone cells [5].

The ability of DFDBA to be osteoconductive and osteoinductive would be influenced by various factors, such as the age of the donor (best between 41 and 50 years old for a man and 51 and 60 years old for a woman), the size of the particles (which must be between 500 and 710 μm to ensure an optimal effect), the residual calcium level (osteo-induction is optimal when the percentage of residual calcium is 2%) [6], as well as the methods of preparation, sterilization, and conservation [7]. It was shown that there is a large variation in the amounts of proteins extracted within different batches of DFDBA, and the authors hypothesized that proteins could be degraded within certain DFDBA batches or present in too small quantity within the bone matrix and therefore remain undetectable with their method [5].

3. Adjuvants to surgery: autologous platelet concentrates

The purpose of using autologous platelet concentrates (PRP and PRF) in oral and implant surgery is to accelerate and improve the phenomena leading to healing, and in particular during surgical procedures aimed at bone regeneration (for review, see [8]).

Platelet-Rich Plasma (PRP), introduced by Marx et al. in 1998, is obtained following two successive centrifugations in tubes with the anticoagulant citrate dextrose A (avoiding platelet activation and degranulation). Gelation of the platelet concentrate is achieved instantly by adding bovine thrombin, recombinant human thrombin, or recombinant human tissue factor, which triggers platelet activation and fibrin polymerization [9].

Authors have developed a simplified protocol to obtain an autologous platelet concentrate without the use of anticoagulants or thrombin called PRF (Platelet-Rich Fibrin) [10]. Venous blood collected without the addition of anticoagulant is immediately centrifuged for 10–12 minutes at 2700–3000 rpm. The authors obtained three layers successively from the bottom to the surface of the tube: the red blood cells, the PRF clot rich in platelets, and on the surface the acellular plasma rich in fibrin.

The natural coagulation mechanism is triggered when blood comes into contact with the surface of the glass tube and allows the production of a fibrin clot rich in platelets and white blood cells, without biochemical changes, that is without the addition of anticoagulant, thrombin or calcium chloride. PRF can be used in the form of gel or membranes.

Platelet-rich fibrin (PRF) has the advantage over PRP of being completely autologous and has been shown to release platelet growth factors over a period of at least one week [11], unlike PRP that releases them within 1 hour following its preparation [12]. Due to the ease of obtaining it, its purely autologous nature, and the fact that the coagulation cascade takes place physiologically without the addition of bovine thrombin, PRF is currently tending to replace PRP.

Platelet concentrates contain fibrinogen, cell adhesion molecules (fibrin, fibronectin, and vitronectin) playing a role in cell migration and osteoconduction, and also growth factors such as PDGF (Platelet-Derived Growth Factor), TGF-β, EGF (Epithelial Growth Factor), IGF (Insulin-like Growth Factor), and VEGF (Vascular Endothelial Growth Factor) [13].

In oral implant surgery, platelet concentrates are used as adjuvants to bone reconstruction procedures. The purpose of their use is to accelerate and improve the phenomena leading to healing, and in particular to the integration of bone grafts and bone regeneration [13].

They are used in many clinical applications: maxillary sinus filling, alveolar bone crest augmentation, mandibular reconstructions, treatment of periodontal pockets, filling of post-extraction dental sockets, and osseointegration of dental implants [14–17]. Studies have been able to show the beneficial effects of platelet concentrates such as improved soft tissue healing [18, 19]. However, the improvement of bone regeneration thanks to the contribution of platelet concentrates is still controversial [20, 21]. Lack of standardization in procurement protocols of these platelet concentrates may explain the lack of concordance in the various studies, and in addition, the kinetics of delivery of growth factors is a mechanism that is still poorly understood, and which may show large variations between patients and in the same patient according to the time of day when blood collection takes place (there are circadian variations in platelet concentration) [10, 11]. In addition, the contradictory results noted in the literature concerning the benefits provided by the use of platelet coagulation factors can be partly explained by the fact that these results come from clinical studies for some and from animal studies for others, and that it is difficult to extrapolate the results obtained from one species to another [22, 23].

On the other hand, the minimum concentration of platelets necessary to obtain a blood clot entering into the criteria defining the PRF is not well specified by the authors. However, they agree on the fact that a clinical benefit can be obtained for a platelet concentration of 1 million/μl of plasma (4 to 7 times the basal level) [24].

4. Use of a combination of particulate allograft (DFDBA) and platelet concentrates (PRF) in oral and maxillo-facial surgery

In our department, we routinely use a combination of particulate allograft (DFDBA 300–500 μm) and platelet concentrates (PRF) for the preservation of alveolar bone volume after dental extractions, for sinus grafts (sinus lifts), and for horizontal and vertical bone grafts.

The DFDBA comes from the cortical part of the long bones of the lower limbs of deceased tissue donors in the Erasmus Hospital Bone and Tissue Bank. It is collected by the Erasmus Bone and Tissue Bank team. The samples are then demineralized in HCl to obtain a residual calcium value <10%. Sterilization is then performed using two chemical baths of NaOH and H_20_2 validated by the Institut Pasteur for the destruction of bacteria and viruses and finally undergoes Gamma 25 kGy irradiation at the end of the process. The different particle sizes are obtained by sieving.

To assess whether this DFDBA and PRF mixture was favorable for post-extraction bone filling, we conducted clinical and histological/histomorphometric research.

First, a retrospective radiological clinical study was conducted on 56 patients for whom 95 extractions had been done, to evaluate vertical alveolar bone loss 3 months after tooth extraction, to find out if a combination of particulate allograft (300–500 μm) and PRF could be beneficial for the patient, with predictable results, to preserve alveolar bone volume. Three months after tooth extraction, the mean of vertical loss of the midbuccal bone wall was 0.72 (SD 0.71) mm (5.53%), indicating a good potential for the technique using DFDBA 300–500 μm and platelet concentrates in alveolar bone preservation [25].

In a second study [26], a retrospective clinical study was performed. A total of 84 patients were included with 247 dental implants, to compare peri-implant bone loss at implants placed in alveolar sockets filled with a particulate allogenous bone graft (DFDBA 300–500 μm) and platelet concentrates *versus* at implants placed in the native bone. At 6 and 12 months, the peri-implant bone loss in sockets preserved with DFDBA and platelet concentrates was similar to the peri-implant bone loss in native bone.

In a recent study [27] to evaluate the bone quality of sinus and alveolar grafts following filling with particulate allogenous bone (DFDBA 300–500 μm) and platelet concentrate (PRF), we realized a prospective interventional clinical and histomorphometric study. A total of 40 bone cores, 2 mm in diameter, were taken from 21 patients: 22 from grafted alveoli, 7 from grafted sinus sites, and 11 from native bone used as a control. Fixed, paraffin-embedded samples were subjected to histological staining with hematoxylin–eosin and Masson's trichrome. Bone maturity of the samples was evaluated by two independent operators using histomorphometric analysis. There existed a greater proportion of lamellar neoformed bone than woven neoformed bone as the healing time increased. Moreover, there was also an increasing proportion of newly formed bone in the grafted sockets as a function of healing time (average: 41.22% ≤ 5 months, 55.89% ˃ 5 months). Resorption of DFDBA particles also appears to be correlated with healing time in the grafted socket (average: 15.43% ≤ 5 months, 13.72% ˃ 5 months). We were able to conclude that performing sinus lift and alveolar socket preservation techniques using DFDBA and PRF results in high-quality, mature bone tissue according to histological criteria.

Our studies show that the use of particulate DFDBA mixed with platelet concentrate (PRF) leads to good clinical results with regard to post-extraction bone preservation and success rate of implants placed in the grafted bone. Moreover, a histomorphometric study shows that this technique results in a high-quality mature bone according to histological criteria.

4.1 Horizontal and vertical bone grafting

For bone grafting of the maxillas, autologous bone grafting has long been considered the gold standard owing to its osteogenic, osteoconductive, and osteoinductive properties [28]. However, this graft, which is taken from intra- or extraoral donor sites, limits the amount of bone available and requires a second invasive surgical procedure, thus increasing the risk of post-operative morbidity [29]. Moreover, it features a mean resorption rate of 50% [28].

Demineralized freeze-dried bone allograft (DFDBA) in the particulate form has been used successfully for many years in the Stomatology and Maxillofacial Surgery Department of the Erasmus Hospital for bone grafting procedures in maxillo-facial and implant surgery.

Its particulate character (particles whose diameter is between 300 and 500 μm and 500–1000 μm) allows its easy adaptation to the recipient bone bed. Nevertheless, the forces applied by the soft tissues can compromise its stability and the maintenance of the volume of the graft, and it is necessary to add a mechanical means of maintenance of volume during the integration period of the bone graft.

The principle of guided bone regeneration (GBR) consists in placing the graft material under a support acting as a space maintainer, to prevent the non-osteogenic tissues from interfering with bone regeneration [30].

To this end, the use of titanium osteosynthesis screws arranged as a "tent peg" is currently considered an effective therapeutic procedure in the treatment of significant vertical bone deficits (**Figure 1**) [31].

We recently performed a 2-year clinical prospective study [submitted] to quantify the study of horizontal oral bone ridge augmentation using GBR with an association of particulate allografts mixed with platelet-rich fibrin, collagen membrane, and tenting screws. This study aimed to radiologically evaluate the horizontal bone gain. A total of 42 patients with an insufficient alveolar bone width for dental implant placement were treated with a GBR technique using a mixture of particulate allograft (demineralized freeze-dried bone allograft 300–500 and 500–1000 μm), advanced platelet-rich fibrin (A-PRF), resorbable collagen membranes, and screw tents (1.2 mm in diameter). Bone gains were measured by cone-beam computed tomography (CBCT) at 9.1 ± 2.0 months post-operatively. A significant mean increase ($P < 0.001$) of 3.2 ± 0.9 mm was observed regardless of bone defect location and without complications during the entire post-operative follow-up. All patients benefited from implant placement following the bone augmentation protocol.

We were able to conclude that maxillomandibular bone augmentation in the horizontal plane by the guided bone regeneration technique using a mixture of particulate allograft, platelet concentrates (A-PRF), and screw-tent in combination with a flap closure technique tension-free mucoperiosteal was a procedure that provides reliable, predictable, and reproducible clinical results. This guided bone regeneration technique differs from previous studies on the subject by its qualitative aspects. Indeed, it is easy to use, considerably reducing operating time, with a low complication rate and an absence of morbidity associated with the donor site in the context of autologous bone harvesting. In addition, all the materials and methods used in the context of this technique are reimbursed for the patient.

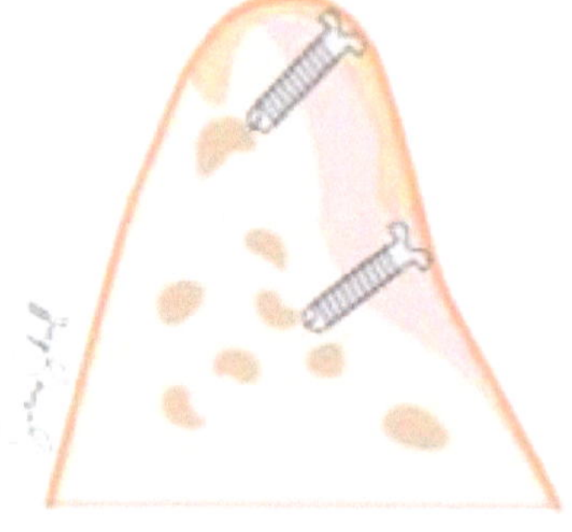

Figure 1.
The placement of osteosynthesis screws arranged in a "tent peg" to counter the forces exerted by the soft tissues. After placement of the demineralized freeze-dried bone allograft (DFDBA) and platelet-rich fibrin (PRF) mixture against the recipient bone bed, a collagenic membrane is positioned to cover the graft. The mucosal flap can be put back in place with sutures.

4.1.1 Clinical case: Horizontal bone grafting

This 51-year-old woman, totally edentulous at the maxilla, presents with significant horizontal bone resorption of the upper jaw (Class IV by Cawood et al. [32]). She wants an implant-supported rehabilitation solution, and it is necessary to perform bone reconstruction before placing implants (**Figure 2**).

Computed tomography (CT) scan in left (B) and right (C) premolar areas shows important horizontal loss of the maxillary bone (**Figures 3–6**).

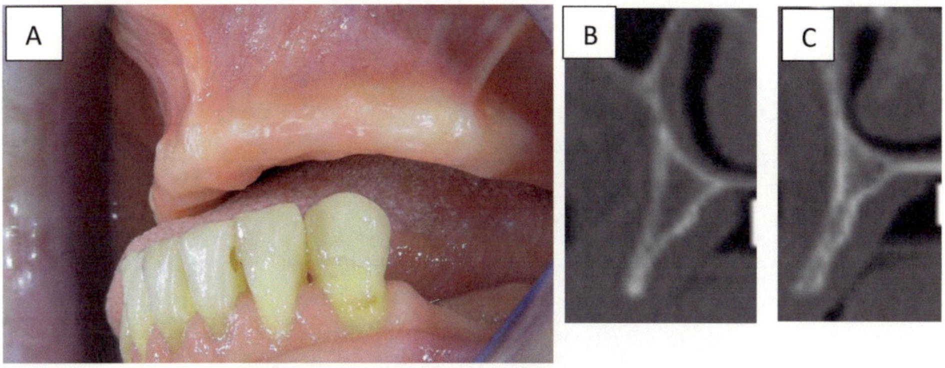

Figure 2.
Intrabuccal clinical view (A) showing horizontal bone resorption of the maxilla.

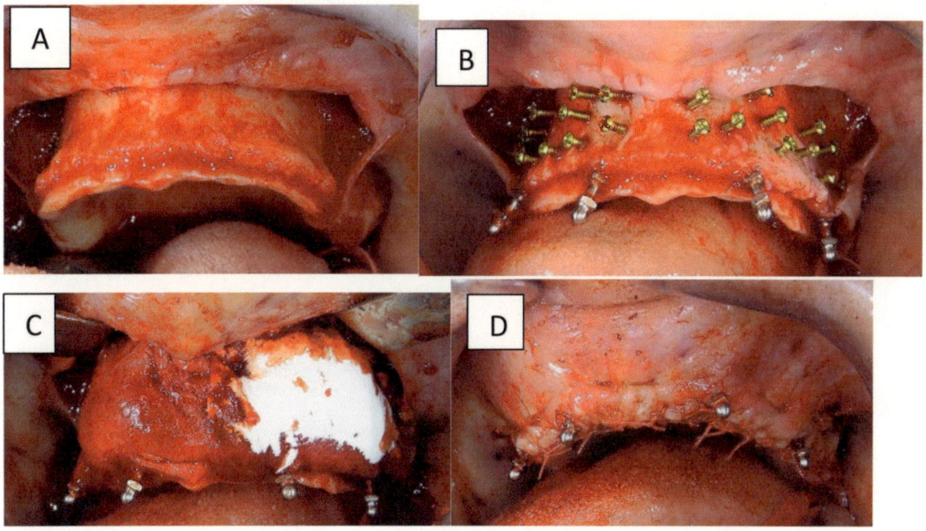

Figure 3.
Surgical procedure. A mucoperiosteal incision is made (A) and a mucoperiosteal flap is released. Screws (1.2 mm diameter) are placed (B), to allow guided bone regeneration and four temporary implants are placed avoid prosthesis pressure on the grafted site. A mix of particulate allograft (demineralized freeze-dried bone allograft (DFDBA) 300–500 μm) and platelet concentrate (platelet-rich fibrin (PRF)) is applied between the screws, in tied contact with bone, and covered with a collagen membrane then by PRF membranes (C). Flap is sutured in place without any tension (D).

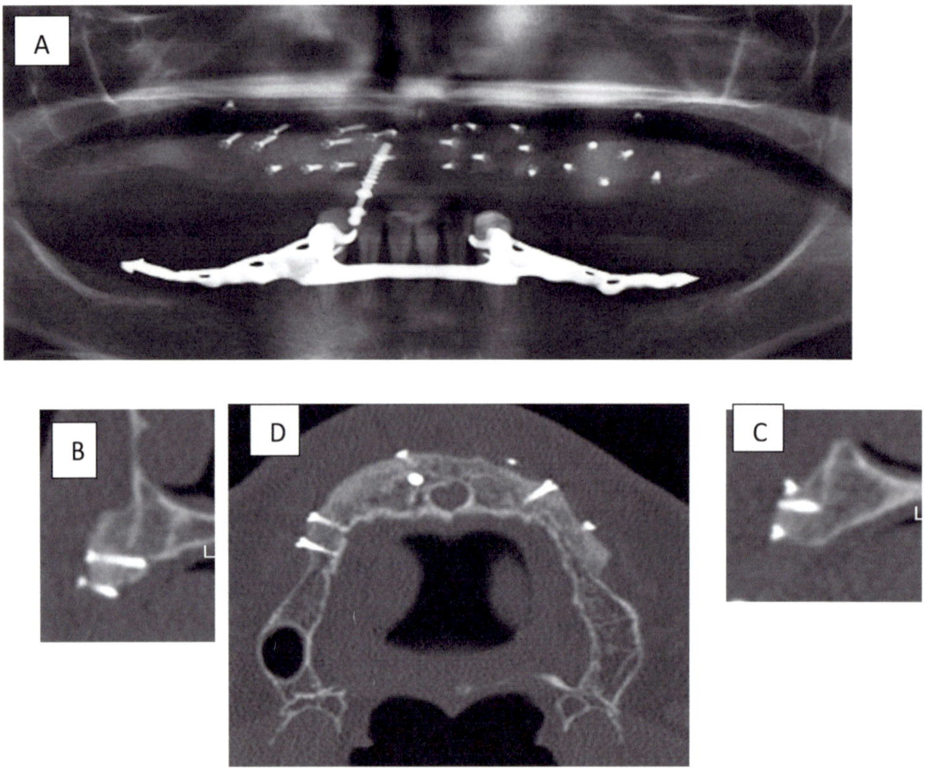

Figure 4.
Radiological assessment 9 months later. The panoramic X-ray (A) and the computed tomography (CT) scan in right premolar (B), left premolar (C), and anterior (D) areas show a bone gain of between 4 and 5 mm over the entire area that has been grafted.

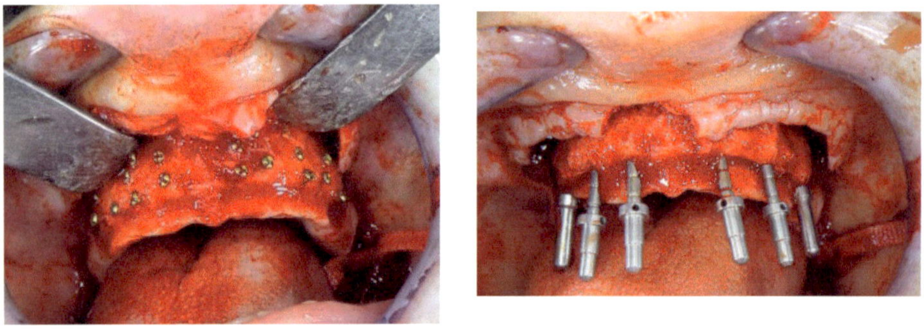

Figure 5.
The placement of six implants 9 months after the grafting procedure, together with removal of tenting screws.

4.1.2 Clinical case: Vertical bone grafting

This 31-year-old woman underwent exeresis of a myxoma of the anterior part of the maxilla 9 years ago. Consecutively, she had lost a part of anterior maxilla, as well as teeth 11, 12, and 13. Clinically, there is a vertical bone loss, together with retracted scar gingiva (**Figures 7–11**).

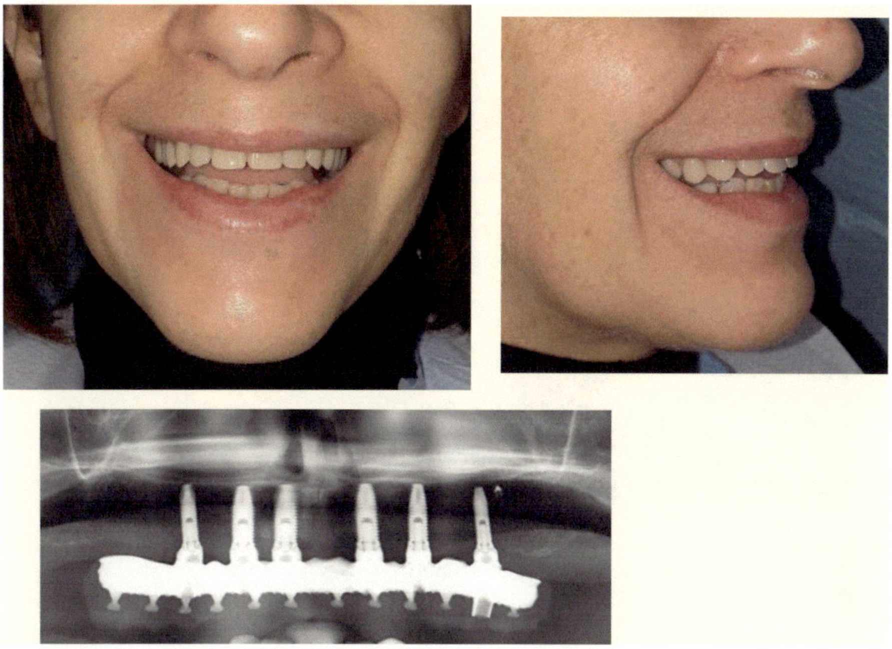

Figure 6.
The final prosthetic result. Six months after the placement of implants, the patient can be provided with a fixed upper bridge screwed on implants.

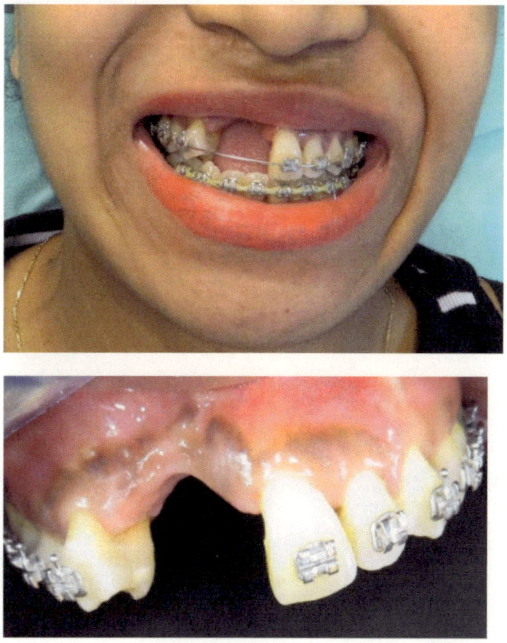

Figure 7.
Clinical view showing vertical bone loss in the area where a myxoma of the anterior part of the maxilla had been removed 9 years ago.

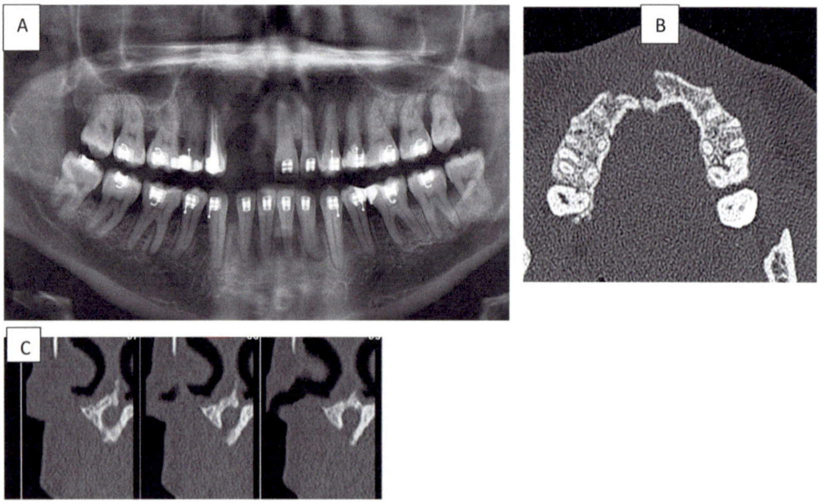

Figure 8.
Panoramic X-ray (A) and computed tomography (CT)-scan axial (B) and sagittal (C) views show the voluminous loss of bone in the anterior region of the maxilla.

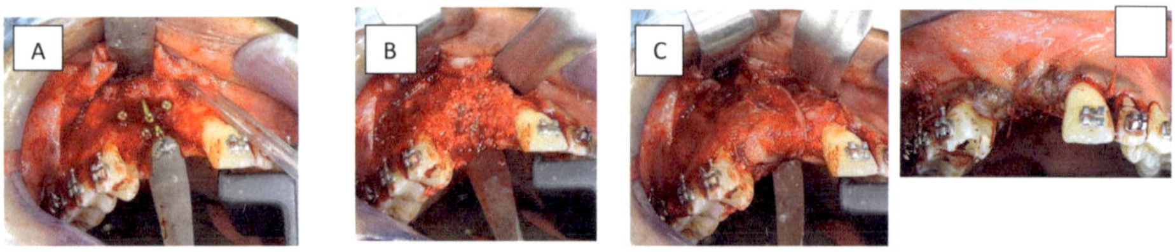

Figure 9.
The day of bone reconstruction, a mucoperiosteal flap is raised, then 1.2 mm screws are placed (A), then a mixing of particulate demineralized freeze-dried bone allograft (DFDBA) 300–500 and 500–1000 (2/1)/platelet-rich fibrin (PRF) are compacted against the recipient bone bed (B), the PRF membranes are placed to cover the graft (C), and the site is sutured together with anterior shift of gingival papillas (D).

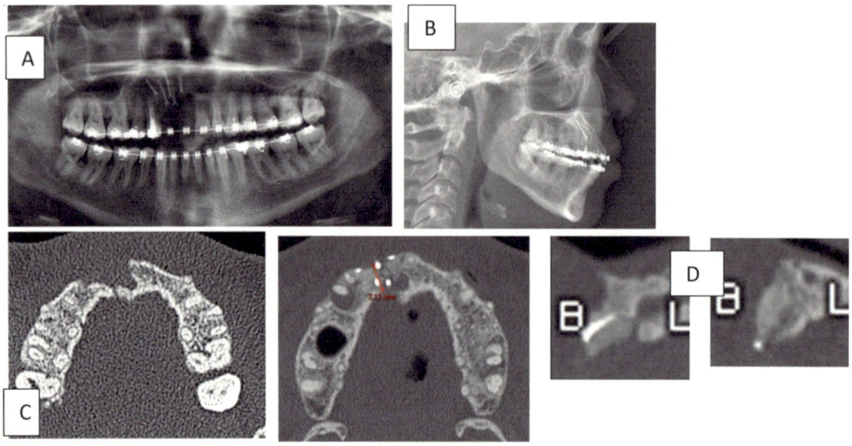

Figure 10.
Nine months later, X-ray assessment: Panoramic X-ray (A), cephalometric R-ray (B), and computed tomography (CT) scan in axial (C) and sagittal (D) views show a good bone reconstruction in the grafted area.

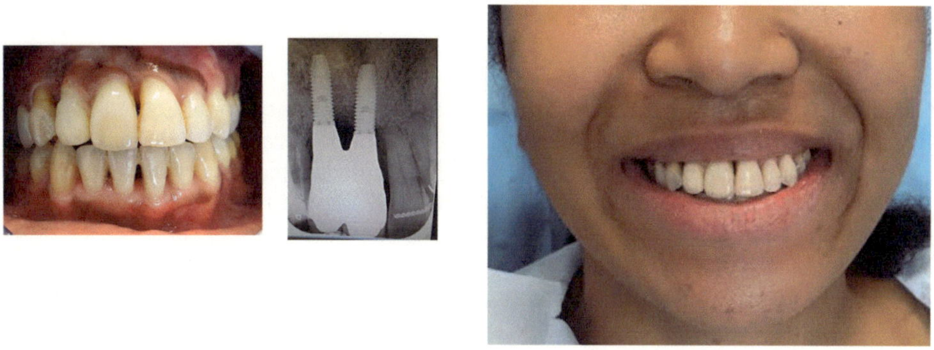

Figure 11.
Two implants could be placed into the bone graft, and the patient was provided with a fixed bridge screwed on implants.

5. Conclusion

Particulate allografts are commonly used in oral and maxillo-facial surgery.

Particulate Demineralized Freeze Dried Bone Allograft (DFDBA) is mainly used in a granulometry 300–500 μm. Mixed with platelet concentrates, it is a material that is easy to handle and to mold in place on bone beds.

Clinical and histomorphometric studies carried out by our team show that the use of this DFDBA and PRF combination gives good results for post-extraction bone volume conservation, maxillary sinus grafts, horizontal and vertical maxillary augmentations.

Conflict of interest

The author declares no conflict of interest.

Author details

Laurence Evrard
Oral and Maxillofacial Surgery Department, Hôpital Universitaire de Bruxelles (HUB), Université libre de Bruxelles, Belgium

*Address all correspondence to: laurence.evrard@hubruxelles.be

References

[1] Bader H. Immediate extraction site grafting: Materials and clinical objectives. Dentistry Today. 2005;**24**(7):86-89 quiz 89

[2] Tischler M, Misch CE. Extraction site bone grafting in general dentistry. Review of applications and principles. Dentistry Today. 2004;**23**(5):108-113

[3] Holtzclaw D, Toscano N, Eisenlohr L, Callan D. The safety of bone allografts used in dentistry: A review. Journal of the American Dental Association (1939). 2008;**139**(9):1192-1199 Review

[4] Zhang M, Powers RM, Wolfinbarger L Jr. Effects of the demineralization process on the osteoinductivity of demineralized bone matrix. Journal of Periodontology. 1997;**68**:1085-1092

[5] Li H, Pujic Z, Xiao Y, Bartold PM. Identification of bone morphogenetic proteins 2 and 4 in commercial demineralized freeze-dried bone allograft preparations: Pilot study. Clinical Implant Dentistry and Related Research. 2000;**2**(2):110-117

[6] Ghanbari Moeintaghavi A, Sargolzaei N, Foroozanfar A, Dadpour Y. Comparative study of Algipore and decalcified freeze-dried bone allograft in open maxillary sinus elevation using piezoelectric surgery. Journal of Advanced Periodontology & Implant Dentistry. 2013;**5**(1):1-6

[7] Schwartz Z, Mellonig JT, Carnes DL, de La Fontaine J, Cochran DL, Dean BB, et al. Ability of commercial demineralized freeze-dried bone allografts. Journal of Periodontology. 1996;**67**:918-926

[8] Bayens M, Glineur R, Evrard L. The use of platelet concentrates: Platelet-rich plasma (PRP) and platelet-rich fibrin (PRF) in bone reconstruction prior to dental implant surgery. Revue Médicale de Bruxelles. 2010;**31**:521-527

[9] Marx RE, Carlson ER, Eichstaedt RM, Schimmele SR, Strauss JE, Georgeff KR. Platelet-rich plasma: Growth factor enhancement for bone grafts. Oral Surgery, Oral Medicine, Oral Pathology, Oral Radiology, and Endodontics. 1998;**85**:638-646

[10] Dohan DM, Choukroun J, Diss A, Dohan SL, Dohan AJ, Mouhyi J, et al. Platelet-rich fibrin (PRF): A second-generation platelet concentrate. Part I: Technological concepts and evolution. Oral Surgery, Oral Medicine, Oral Pathology, Oral Radiology, and Endodontics. 2006;**101**:37-44

[11] Dohan DM, Choukroun J, Diss A, Dohan SL, Dohan AJ, Mouhyi J, et al. Platelet-rich fibrin (PRF): A second-generation platelet concentrate. Part II: Platelet-related biologic features. Oral Surgery, Oral Medicine, Oral Pathology, Oral Radiology, and Endodontics. 2006;**101**:45-50

[12] Hallman M, Thor A. Bone substitutes and growth factors as an alternative/complement to autogenous bone for grafting in implant dentistry. Periodontology 2000. 2008;**47**:172-192 Review

[13] Marx RE, Garg AK. Dental and Craniofacial Applications of Platelet-Rich Plasma. US-Michigan: Quintessence Publishing Co, Inc.; 2005

[14] Steigmann M, Garg AK. A comparative study of bilateral sinus lifts performed with platelet-rich plasma alone versus alloplastic graft material

reconstituted with blood. Implant Dentistry. 2005;**14**:261-266

[15] Ito K, Yamada Y, Naiki T, Ueda M. Simultaneous implant placement and bone regeneration around dental implants using tissue-engineered bone with fibrin glue, mesenchymal stem cells and platelet-rich plasma. Clinical Oral Implants Research. 2006;**17**:579-586

[16] Hanna R, Trejo PM, Weltman RL. Treatment of intrabony defects with bovine-derived xenograft alone and in combination with platelet-rich plasma: A randomized clinical trial. Journal of Periodontology. 2004;**75**:1668-1677

[17] Anitua E, Orive G, Aguirre JJ, Andía I. Clinical outcome of immediately loaded dental implants bioactivated with plasma rich in growth factors: A 5-year retrospective study. Journal of Periodontology. 2008;**79**:1168-1176

[18] Choukroun J, Diss A, Simonpieri A, Girard MO, Schoeffler C, Dohan SL, et al. Platelet-rich fibrin (PRF): A second-generation platelet concentrate part IV: Clinical effects on tissue healing. Oral Surgery, Oral Medicine, Oral Pathology, Oral Radiology, and Endodontics. 2006;**101**(3):e56-e60

[19] Hom DB, Linzie BM, Huang TC. The healing effects of autologous platelet gel on acute human skin wounds. Archives of Facial Plastic Surgery. 2007;**9**(3):174-183

[20] Piemontese M, Aspriello SD, Rubini C, Ferrante L, Procaccini M. Treatment of periodontal intrabony defects with demineralized freeze-dried bone allograft in combination with platelet-rich plasma: A comparative clinical trial. Journal of Periodontology. 2008;**79**(5):802-810

[21] Singh A, Kohli M, Gupta N. Platelet rich fibrin: A novel approach for osseous regeneration. The Journal of Maxillofacial and Oral Surgery. 2012;**11**(4):430-434

[22] Casati MZ, de Vasconcelos Gurgel BC, Gonçalves PF, Pimentel SP, da Rocha Nogueira Filho G, Nociti FH Jr, et al. Platelet-rich plasma does not improve bone regeneration around peri-implant bone defects--a pilot study in dogs. International Journal of Oral and Maxillofacial Surgery. 2007;**36**:132-136

[23] Gürbüzer B, Pikdöken L, Urhan M, Süer BT, Narin Y. Scintigraphic evaluation of early osteoblastic activity in extraction sockets treated with platelet-rich plasma. Journal of Oral and Maxillofacial Surgery. 2008;**66**:2454-2460

[24] Weibrich G, Hansen T, Kleis W, Buch R, Hitzler WE. Effect of platelet concentration in platelet-rich plasma on peri-implant bone regeneration. Bone. 2004;**34**:665-671

[25] Baniasadi B, Evrard L. Alveolar ridge preservation after tooth extraction with DFDBA and platelet concentrates: A radiographic retrospective study. The Open Dentistry Journal. 2017;**11**:99-108

[26] Bui Qoc J, Vang A, Evrard L. Peri-implant bone loss at implants placed in preserved alveolar bone versus implants placed in native bone: A retrospective radiographic study. The Open Dentistry Journal. 2018;**12**:529-545

[27] Wardani A, Tran B, Duterre M, Larabi I, Waskiewicz K, Louryan S, et al. Healing of particulate allografts mixed with platelet concentrates in ridge preservation and sinus lift: A prospective histomorphometric study. Morphologie. 28 Mar 2023:S1286-0115(23)00027-9. DOI: 10.1016/j.morpho.2023.03.001 [Online ahead of print]

[28] Von Arx T, Buser D. Horizontal ridge augmentation using autogenous block

grafts and the guided bone regeneration technique with collagen membranes: A clinical study with 42 patients. Clinical Oral Implants Research. 2006;**17**:359-366

[29] Nkenke E, Schultze-Mosgau S, Radespiel-Tröger M, Kloss F, Neukam FW. Morbidity of harvesting of chin grafts: A prospective study. Clinical Oral Implants Research. 2001;**12**:495-502

[30] Wang HL, Boyapati L. "PASS" principles for predictable bone regeneration. Implant Dentistry. 2006;**15**:8-17

[31] Borie G, Naman E, Vincent-Bugnas S. Screw tenting with fast system® and allograft plus i. PRF® in guided bone regeneration–case series. Clinical Oral Implants Research. 2019;**30**:421-421

[32] Cawood J, Howell RA. Reconstructive preprosthetic surgery. I. Anatomical considerations. International Journal of Oral and Maxillofacial Surgery. 1991;**20**(2):75-82